Cor

Contents

Once we felt safe ...

... we could begin to explore...

Sex, drugs and...

The long haul...

Come on over, we're just next door

Pick a card, any card, pick it from the top

... and now for something completely different ...

Appendices

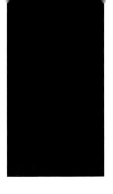

Foreword

I am sure the reader will be impressed by the honesty, courage and overall, the compassion expressed in these pages. It is to the credit of the team manager and staff that such an ethos is fostered. The emphasis on individual difference and respecting the individuality of the men, attempting to look beyond their particular symptoms and behaviours, to see the person often hidden within, is a huge part of the success of the team, and much of the reason why the unit seems like home.

A reflective practice group for the staff was set up to facilitate this 'looking beyond' the symptoms and behaviours, in an attempt to understand what might be going on in the men's internal worlds, how previous experiences and fears may be played out on the unit and with staff, and to recognise what staff may be bringing from their own experiences and fears. I have been honoured to be part of this group and applaud the courage of those who have attended, particularly John for being able to express his own doubts and anxieties, allowing a safe place for others to explore their own. To be able to hold such doubts and uncertainties, without flight into the safety of 'certainty' and 'knowing', can feel quite risky, especially in an age of increasingly diagnosis-led and rigidly targeted treatments which often ignore the complexity of the individual. Expressing doubts and uncertainties, however uncomfortable, enables productive and constructive debate, leading to creative and flexible thinking, in which different perspectives can be examined.

In such an atmosphere 'risk' can better be tolerated and managed. To attempt to understand, even in small part, how someone may have arrived at where they are, for how their experiences may have shaped and influenced their behaviour, does not mean excusing it, but rather enables a means of dealing with it more productively. The behaviour may be just as problematic, but by being understood, it can be viewed more compassionately, and the individual helped to change.

One story particularly for me demonstrates the care and effort made to retain a sense of the individual's identity and that was with a man who was relapsing into more severe illness.

The staff were trying to keep him on the unit, where he felt safe, but this was becoming increasingly difficult. He was in seclusion with a member of staff outside. In the midst of his distress he put his hand up to the window in the door, and the member of staff put hers up to meet his on the other side of the glass.

Such a moment of intimacy and compassion, in what must have been a frightening episode for both patient and staff, is hard to measure.

Dr Vanessa J Griffiths,
Consultant Clinical Psychologist

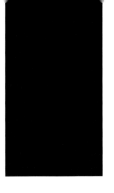

Introduction

This book is about a low secure unit (LSU) in Cornwall. I didn't actually know what a low secure unit was to start with. When I did, I was more than a little nervous. However, I actually arrived, and what impressed me was how warm and home-like it was and how safe I felt. I was genuinely surprised.

One of the men had been quite disturbed overnight and had continued to be so that morning. He was pacing up and down, gesticulating, shouting and threatening staff. I suggested some additional medication. One of the staff, gently replied to me we try not to use medication here; we like to talk to the men. Wow!

Here was a place that wanted to work with people without immediately reaching for medication. Again and again I noticed things were being done differently than what I had experienced previously. I would often comment and ask how the staff had managed specific situations; how they had created a safe and homely feel amongst a complex population. The staff were often bewildered at my question or shrugged their shoulders commenting they had never really thought about it, we just do it. As I persisted, the staff began to realise maybe they were doing something differently and something that might be worth describing.

This is not a text book, nor is it a series of references. Instead it is a collection of stories about people and about clinical situations other low secure units may also experience. It is written in a style which might be suitable for the men who we see and to whom we may offer a place, and their families in order that they too may get a sense of their son's environment. We believe it will be useful to staff who work on other low secure units who, unable to visit Cornwall, want to have a sense of what happens down in the South West. We also hope it becomes of interest to students from the humanities who are curious about the person in their work, and who may wonder about what it is like on a modern psychiatric unit.

The book reflects real clinical practice at the tin face, both good and bad, rather than being a description of 'this is how it should be done'. We don't know how it should be done. We're doing it as we are doing it, learning as we go along and are happy to receive suggestions from other units so there may be a broader and shared clinical experience of low secure work. This is the art of psychiatry.

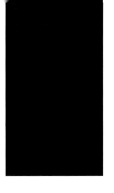

Acknowledgements

Thanks firstly to the men and to the families who contributed. It was a privilege to meet and share part of your lives and to sit with you as we read together those parts of the book written about each of you individually. It was good to laugh together, to be part of your enthusiasm at being included, to take on your comments and corrections and to be intrigued by how you chose your names for the book. Thanks also for signing our consent form.

I am also grateful to Sandra Miles and Vicky Wood for their genuine interest and feel for the work; to Cornwall Partnership NHS Foundation Trust and to Ellen Wilkinson for offering and continuing my job as a locum on the Bowman Unit. A privilege, a great team to work with and such an extraordinary experience that has taught me many things and as a result refined my practice.

We asked a number of people to read our drafts. We particularly want to thank Marg Little and Sarah Fisher whose outstanding commitment, willingness, attention to detail and creativity made it happen. Thanks also to Dawn Spry, Denise Rowe, Angela Rouncefield, Mike Metcalfe, Nick Kitson, John Morgan, Mike Murphy and Bernadette Rheeder for their support.

Finally I want to thank Karen Masters. Karen has been outstanding throughout, typing, re-typing and typing again the various drafts and continuing to do so, despite Iain (who almost deleted the entire book off the computer) Knox, with such good humour. She also makes fantastic pasties! Thank you for your patience and insight.

John Little

one

"Optimism is the key:
naive, unfounded and blind
it may on occasion be, but it
remains essential if clinicians
and their institutions are
not to degenerate into
instruments of repression".

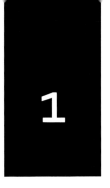

1 Where's Cornwall?

A few years ago, while browsing through a psychiatric journal I came across a story of a psychiatrist who had described his year in Cornwall. It sounded magical and we decided to go for a family adventure. We took the boys, Alex and Robbie out of school and Bridgie, sensing the same adventure, came along and we headed for Bodmin.

Two or three years later we met the author of the article and said thanks. Five years later we have returned as have all of our children, both with us and separately, having made what we hope is a lifelong friendship with the people and the county.

Cornwall is a slender county that dips its toe into the Atlantic. As with other Celtic regions of the UK, there is something mystical about Cornwall. It is both maritime and rural. As such the community is close knit with small villages dotted across a stunning landscape. People tend to know one another and are aware of the old psychiatric hospital, St Lawrence, and the prison, both of which were in Bodmin.

Michaela was born and bred in Bodmin. She has

devoted her life to working with people with mental illness having started as a healthcare assistant (HCA). When she left college she wanted to train as a 'proper nurse'. However her dad became unwell and so she stayed. Thankfully, she was encouraged to apply for registered mental nurse (RMN) training.

She worked on the first ward to be moved from the large St Lawrence Asylum into the community and opened the first supported domestic house (SDH) for the Trust in Lostwithiel. She then spent some years as a community psychiatric nurse (CPN) before being selected as the manager for Selwood House and then Bowman Low Secure Unit. Alongside this she expressed an interest in the whole life philosophy; the Trust being a pilot site for this initiative. This enabled Michaela to meet representatives from the World Health Organisation and with this, came the opportunity to develop rehabilitation services in Palestine and Italy.

She lives on a property in rural Cornwall with her lovely and equally talented daughter Cassie and walked for two hours to get to work when the roads were blocked by snow! Here's her view. It's important as this book is really about Michaela, her vision and her drive.

Michaela

Following my interview, I was both shocked and pleasantly surprised when I received the phone call informing me I had been successful in obtaining the role of manager for a new low secure unit. Having a background in rehabilitation and recovery and only having worked with clients detained by the Ministry of Justice in an open environment, (very successfully!) I wondered why me? I must have said something right to get the job!

Over the next few days anxiety began to set in, how was I going to lead a team in an area that was quite alien to me? Could I live up to everyone's expectation? How could I ensure it would be a success?I re-looked at my interview presentation - 'How I saw the unit developing within the first 12 months and why I was the right person for the job!' I remembered the focus of my presentation was 'Doing it Differently' and that was what I set out to achieve. I was determined to provide a service which was innovative, progressive and based on the principles of whole life and social inclusion.

As a new service, I was really lucky and in a prime position – I could hand pick my own team! I was shocked by the sheer number of applications for the vacant posts which came from far and wide. All had a range of experience in different fields of nursing. Besides experience, it was also important to me, to look at what else these individuals could bring to this newly developing team.

With the team in place we commenced a two week training programme. Not only was this important in terms of training staff in the subjects necessary for them, it was also important in terms of team building. It was pleasing to see how well the individuals gelled. Because we all came from different walks of life it was good to have the opportunity to find out about each other and listen to each other's experiences. This time allowed us to share ideas about what we wanted the unit to become. What we never lost sight of during this time was the focus on rehabilitation and recovery.

The clients coming into the unit were introduced, over a period of weeks to allow them time to settle. It also allowed us time to get to know each client as an individual. Too often a person's history comes before them and they are judged even before they arrive. What we have found is the history and the person do not often match!

As clients and staff got to know each other we slowly started to introduce the principles of whole life and social inclusion into the unit. To implement this philosophy within the NHS often requires 'thinking outside the box' in order to make things happen for individuals.

Taking the time to find out what might help an individual is a way of engaging with them before undertaking more in depth work. Clinicians do not always have high expectations of clients and clients do not have high expectations of themselves. Therefore helping clients work towards their hopes, dreams and aspirations is very important. In order to 'think outside the box' and work with clients to help them reach their hopes and dreams a certain amount of positive risk taking needs to happen, with responsibility given back to the client. This has not always worked as the client may not have been ready at that particular time. We then have to revisit the situation and try again.

Michaela by Jess

I've been putting off writing my piece for a while now, waiting for the inspiration and taking time to think and reflect on what it is about Bowman that makes it special and different from any other place I've worked before.

Prior to commencing my post, I had started getting second thoughts, Cornwall had never had a low secure unit (LSU) before and I didn't know what I was letting myself in for. Of course like anything new, there was a lot of scare mongering amongst staff from other units. Stories of notorious patients with long and often violent histories were rumoured to be going to Bowman. As a fairly newly qualified female nurse I was apprehensive to say the least. What did put my mind at ease was the management which was going to lead the new team of Bowman. I had worked with Michaela at my previous post in an open rehabilitation unit and was comforted by her style of working.

Michaela's philosophy of social inclusion and her gentle non-judgemental approach to the patients, treating them as real human beings who have the needs, desires and feelings we all do. Her style of management makes her so approachable. She will support her colleagues to overcome personal difficulties that may conflict with work arrangements. Her direct but non-threatening approach ensures we all stay focused and deliver the best service we can for the men.

One of the things that makes Bowman so special is the team Michaela picked.

As colleagues we treat each other as close friends, supporting each other in the bad times and celebrating in the good times. I feel this also benefits the guys as we always have a 'united front'. Although some of the guys may try to play one off [staff] against the other it doesn't cause 'team splitting' as we respect each others' decisions and style of working. We don't always agree (otherwise we wouldn't be human), but we are able to be open and honest with each other and discuss like adults our difference of opinions and compromise.

Each low secure unit will be different as each sits in a distinctive social, historical and geographic context. Cornwall is a small community with a mystic heritage and these elements are an important feature of our practice. A person of Michaela's experience is also difficult to replicate. However we also feel the philosophy of care offered on Bowman can be applied to other units.

Why am I locked up?

I don't think I have schotrania truthfully ~~as~~ the illness is because of drugs that have damaged the health

I wan't to be able to go out when I wan't to at night and during the day
I wan't to be able to drink alcahol because it helps me and its not illegal

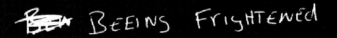 BEEING FRIGHTENED

Food

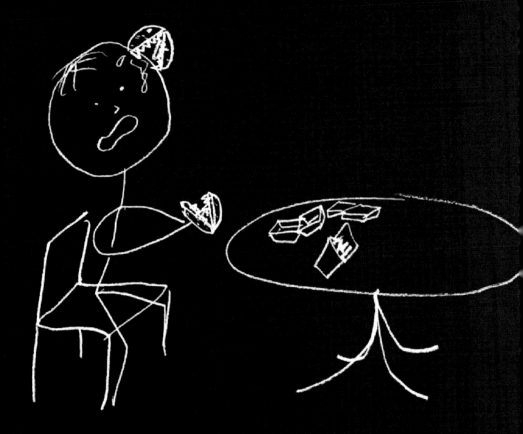

*1. Sausage egg chips

Fatty

D/Y+ (clue)

* Fatty

The appearance of a fried
fatty meal to me desn't
appeal to be correct

Answer

FATTY

Being lonely and frightened

When my family visiting no one out side

Moving on

I have decided that the purchase of alcohol is detrimental of my health, No purchase of % Alcohol will be made.

£50.00

INCOME

Income	out
Week 2 £180	£49.00 P/Accoums
	131.00

£131.00
Tabacco ⨯ 14 packs?

12.5g   25g   50g
  1   2   4

12.5g = £3.00
25.g = £6.00
50g = £11.00

50g = 4° ⨯ 11 £44

4° = 4 days
    4 ⨯ £4 16

£40.00 TABACCO

Making it...

Dear doctor little
please tell me why im being keapt for
So long as I dont see why I should
be locked up because im not a criminal
or a gonerment agent and im not mentally
ill at the moment, why should it take
a long tiome when I dont want to be
here

Dir sir or madam

I wish to complain that since I was first sectioned and put on clopixol I have had the following symtons almost constantly for 4½ years – erectile dysfunctic, impotence lose of feeling in my penis, difficulty maintaining an erection and difficulty getting one. I have also had these problems on slaripine on clopixol which I was on for 2½ years I had ocular gyric crisises, tremors, massive sedation and resportory difficultys

yours faithfuly

I wish you would stop
making me feel crap. when
I've always wanted to have
a heart of gold. which I do
but I've had rape issues for
years thinking somone out
there made me through
hypnosis or brain washing
have sex with a dog. which
made me vident!

To All staff and
Doctors ect

Merry Christmas

Let me go. stop beeing
the way you are to
me

I went home today. It was really good I wish i had more time. I saw my mums giant rabbit and saw her dogs she has a German shepard and a Jack russle.

today was really good im exited that I've got 4 hours down to pettle and im hoping to move there everything seems to be good and I want to help it that way. I was pleased to hear that I could start going to evening clubs

I enjoyed my home leave today. I went for a walk in the woods with mum and my escorts, cooked a meal; it was very enjoyable I would like more time home and only one escort.

I am feeling fine and am hopefully awaiting a community treatment order or equivalent. I can tell you I am able to identify thoughts that are caused by my illness e.g thinking my life has been led here by corrupt people, which is quite a scary thought but I know this past thought cant be true. and I think that my medication is the best.

Mr A was shortlisted and offered an interview for a job. Sadly he replapsed and was unable to attend on the day.

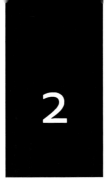

2

Who are our men?

"The attitude of mind... is the whole question. From this everything follows and without it change or humanity or hope is not possible."

Who are our men – a public view

"Insane patients allowed out on day leave". This was a headline from an online Australian tabloid, The Herald Sunday, 6 November 2009. You can imagine how the article unfolded, scant details but those given were sensationalised, and although not necessarily stated, specific judgements were made and advice given. Conversely, psychiatry had sanitised their account with a professional language. The reports were detailed, lengthy, and comprehensive as they itemised and described a series of incidents. Both accounts are true.

Who are our men – a medical view

There is a similarity about a lot of our men. They have had and continue to have, more than their fair share of adversity. Almost without exception, they have come from complicated families with difficult childhoods and limited schooling. Drug abuse is common with marijuana, amphetamines, heroin, ecstasy, solvent abuse and alcohol. If that's not enough, they develop not only schizophrenia, but a treatment resistant schizophrenia. It is this that has often been associated with the series of events which has led them to our unit. At this level they again appear indistinguishable from each other.

Who are our men – a personal view

Laurence believed he had animals inside his body. At the same time as telling us this, he believed he was being told a nurse was entering his bedroom in another part of the building, and cutting off his face, people were biting off his nose and hitting him in the back of his head. He also thought the staff were entering his room at night and murdering him when he wasn't aware.

When Paul went to bed, he was entering a room waist-deep in snakes which tore at his flesh, and spiders that enveloped him with their legs and pinned him to his bed.

Dean describes how his mother wasn't really his mother. The person in front of him was a distorted version of her, speaking to him across time. These experiences continued every day despite our on-going treatment attempts.

Who are our men – a human view

Jono with his cheeky grin, grew up within a family tradition of car boot sales. He continues to wheel and deal like 'Del-boy'. Laurence started off being a journalist. He now spends time carefully painting Napoleonic figurines as a way of distracting himself from his continuous experiences.

Lee, base guitarist, Tom on keyboard (who had also worked as a volunteer in Ghana) and Zach, artist, song writer and lead singer joined together for their recent musical gig in Plymouth and the Bodmin Hospital Fete. They are booked for the South West Rehab Conference and hopefully the Cornwall Partnership NHS Foundation Trust Annual Members' Meeting.

Paul who has a wicked sense of humour and who walks down to Link into Learning twice a week as he attempts to learn to read and write.

Mr A who despite having totalled over a hundred violent incidents had, as a younger man been offered a scholarship for ballet.

Owen had been trialled for Premier League football. I watched him one evening up at the Dragon Centre as he skilfully kicked the ball just over the head of the person in front of him, sped around him and shot the ball into the back of the net. I continued to watch as he passed the ball to a fellow team member who had a better opportunity of scoring. I saw him support and congratulate one of our other men, who after the match was standing back awkwardly.

Tony maintains keen interest in steam trains. Mark watches the stock exchange and was concerned at Kraft's intention to buy out Cadburys.

Despite the 'horror stories' we've found getting to know the person behind the story makes a remarkable difference. It re-connects us with our shared humanity. That's who they are.

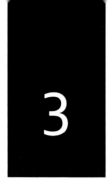

3 Everyone gets frightened

I had worked in Cornwall five years earlier. As our children grew up and left home, my wife and I wanted to return to Cornwall.

I contacted the Trust wondering whether there might be a job. On the phone, Suzanne, one of the most delightful and accommodating people in medical administration I have had the pleasure to work with said she was sure they would be happy to see me back. Some time later I got a follow-up e-mail asking whether or not I would be interested in working in an LSU. I didn't know what an LSU was and read on - the letters stood for low secure unit and then interestingly after that there was the following 'not forensic'. I was struck by the phrase 'not forensic' thinking to myself if it wasn't forensic, why mention it? However the prospect of being able to come to a job and accommodation on the other side of the world was reassuring and I could sort things out once I arrived.

Once in Cornwall I asked a couple of people who I knew from our last visit what low secure units were all about. I knew what I had to do was make an appointment with the Medical Director, Ellen.

Our conversation went along the following lines:

John and Ellen

"I'm a bit nervous!"

Ellen paid me a nice compliment and said she remembered me and saw me as being a safe pair of hands. She explained the usual psychiatrist had been off sick. There had been a few locums and the unit could do with a period of stability. I thanked Ellen for her compliment. I also explained, that although I was a locum and ultimately required to go where I was sent, I didn't want to become trapped in an unfamiliar setting with no prospect of being able to change over to a coastal community mental health team which had been the original plan. She understood and invited me to check in with her over the next three months or sooner, particularly if I had any concerns. Having been able to have an open, honest and direct discussion I felt relieved. I realised I had been frightened.

Paul had become content with his place in hospital. It was warm, home-like and safe. He expressed few symptoms and remained as he had been described in his school records, 'placid, unmotivated but likeable'. Having previously managed people in the community, I was a little bit surprised Paul was still on an inpatient unit and particularly on a low secure unit. Reading through his file and noting his index offence was some 20 years earlier, it still didn't quite make sense. I began to think about Paul moving on, albeit slowly and gradually. Considerable discussion took place with both Paul and his mother, highlighting that whatever change occurred, it needed to occur slowly.

We decided on a six month transition period. There was some initial enthusiasm from Paul and then some more familiar staying in bed. There was some response to gentle persuasion and cajoling and some movement with Fettle House (the open rehabilitation unit) being able to offer Paul a greater range of activities and interests. Around this time, Paul began to describe his abnormal experiences again.

He wondered whether or not the staff were influencing his thoughts and were brain washing him - similar thoughts to those he had had at the time of his index offence. He said he was only agreeing to the move because other people wanted him to move. The team were aware of this and other possible stressors. Paul was about to face another tribunal and likely disappointment and he was in the process of leaving Bowman and moving to Fettle House. His symptoms could be an exacerbation of his illness. We didn't feel there were any drug or alcohol concerns and he had tested negative on random screening. We weren't worried about medication as he was on depot medication and he had not been physically unwell.

We sat with Paul and he began to talk about the unfairness of his situation; of how long he had been in the system, that other people who were violent had been able to move on. It seemed every unit he went to he ended up staying for the longest period of time. He recalled being in Broadmoor where he was up every morning five days a week doing ceramics and how he used to travel around the county on leave with his mother. He felt safe. He now reported he had given up and, he would never be allowed to leave. We had an image of a little boy on his first day at school. Over a series of conversations, Paul was able to acknowledge how frightened he was of being discharged, of being alone and scared of repercussions against his original offence. Like me, Paul was frightened.

The staff were also frightened. While we were aware if we did nothing, nothing would change, others were frightened that if we pushed, we may exacerbate Paul's abnormal experiences and create a situation where he had no other choice other than to attack us or himself. This would secure his stay or begin the process by which he would be returned to the safety of a more secure setting. As a team we could have become divided. Instead we acknowledged the dilemma we were in, accepted different staff had different experiences and it would be unwise to push ahead without all of us being on board. We talked and agreed to slow the move down, share our concerns with Paul and continue to watch. We were able to agree to take a risk by neither increasing his medication nor restricting his leave.

We asked Paul what we should do. Interestingly, Paul, himself recognised the dilemma. He said he knew the staff would panic, and he was able to say he just wanted to stay in one place. He understood he wasn't able to stay on Bowman, and confirmed the fear of others, recalling how he had hit another patient in order to be transferred. Eventually we were able to think about another way of seeing Paul's experiences. The snakes and reptiles which he believed were ripping pieces off him could also be a metaphor for his life. The team were ripping him apart - wanting him to do things he was frightened of doing - namely leaving and moving to another place. Slowly there began to be a subtle change, the team relaxed and Paul began to ask to go to visit Fettle. As a team we had been frightened.

Interestingly Paul returned one day and recounted how he had come across a little boy who had been visiting Fettle House with his family. Paul described how the little boy had come up to him with his hand outstretched and showed him all of his pocket money. I don't know what this meant, but I knew instinctively it was important. I now see it was about trust.

Unexpectedly, other parts of a system which we imagined would routinely accept and support our men also became unnerved once they knew the men had been on a low secure unit.

The manager for a Supported Domestic House (SDH) was careful to involve our team, the Assertive Outreach Team, the Community Mental Health Team and the GP in order to put a robust and consistent package in place for Zach. Cautiously, with a bed kept for Zach on the low secure unit; the Housing Manager insisted on a one month period of daily visits followed by one month of overnight leaves plus one month of full-time leave before his placement was agreed.

To his credit, Ian was able to acknowledge this was the first time they had taken someone with Zach's background. There were teething problems. The staff rang one morning saying their house cat had been acting strangely. They wondered whether Zach had any problems with animals. Initially we were quite taken aback. Then we were able to recall our own experiences of having been frightened when we were uncertain or unfamiliar with someone we were about to meet. In response, our staff went across every day and sat with the house staff to reassure and encourage them to get to know Zach. To appreciate him for who he was as a person rather than remaining stuck with what their fears may have unwittingly created. They did so and Zach is still there two years later. Our colleagues had been frightened.

Nicola and Dean

Nicola had largely tried to bring Dean up by herself. It was difficult. Nicola described him as always being strong minded. It was easy to see how anyone would give in to insistent and at times intimidating demands, particularly as he grew physically into manhood. Perhaps to appease, it was understandable how 'Yes' no longer meant 'Yes' and 'No' no longer meant 'No'.

Dean was settling, and we wanted to offer him opportunities off the unit with his family. Everyone consistently commented he appeared to be better when he was outside. The problem was Nicola wasn't able to tell us if she was frightened to have her son home. He would ring up and demand a visit. We would check with Nicola and then the visit would go ahead. Fortunately, for everyone concerned, Nicola had a good relationship with Debbie, the nurse from the Community Forensic Team. Exhausted, frightened and intimidated both by Dean and by ourselves, Nicola finally revealed to Debbie that at times she found it difficult.

As we began to disentangle the mix up, it seemed what was happening was, Dean would ask for leave; we would check with Nicola who said yes; and Dean went home for increasing periods of time including, eventually overnight leave. When we attempted to clarify and confirm home visits with Nicola she would present cheerfully, saying yes that she wanted Dean home. When we queried this, Dean would angrily turn on us.

Debbie, Nicola, Dean and ourselves all sat down and talked about the difficulties of mixed messages. We tried to seek clarity and decide what might be manageable in the long-term. We wanted to help Nicola to be able to say to Dean, that while she still loved him, he wasn't able to come home as often as he had been. She needed to be able to give this as a clear message herself. She burst into tears and fled the room. Debbie described the considerable previous work she had been done with Nicola, trying to get her to remain clear and consistent. It was striking that when it came to the crunch, she wasn't able to do this. We remained anxious about any further visits because we were never clear what Nicola was actually saying or what was actually going on. We became frightened.

The situation changed. Dean had gradually been allowed unescorted leave in the local area. He absconded, drank and went to his Mum's. We had alerted her and the police and Dean was brought back to the unit. We sat down again and re-negotiated a leave plan. Nicola made a kind gesture to her son and asked us whether or not she could take him out for a coffee after the meeting. It was a lovely gesture and we were all happy to agree. In order to avoid 'getting our wires crossed' Jess clarified it was for the afternoon and not overnight.

Dean suddenly turned on Jess, screamed, and gesticulated with his finger, fixing her with a threatening and intimidating stare. He was barely able to control himself from getting up out of the chair, his fury almost paralysing the room and drawing the attention of the other staff.

I'm not sure what made the difference. It may have been Nicola - having received and largely accepted these tirades as her due, found it unacceptable to see another person subjected to that. At the time, Jess was full of the flu and had come into work because we were short staffed. She barely had the strength to contribute in her usual enthusiastic and committed way. Dean left the room. Nicola said what he had just done was right out of order and unless he apologised, she didn't want to take him for coffee. For the first time Nicola and the clinical team were united. We had all been frightened.

We have tried to encourage different teams to come and meet the men so they can get an understanding of the unit and how the person presents having been with us for some time. Many have done so. Mark, a Community Support Worker, made an outstanding effort. Coming regularly, engaging with Mr A, (his preferred name for this book), taking him out to his flat and supporting him. Staff from Pentree Residential Care Home where Tony had been discharged to, were invited to the unit as he was recovering from a further manic phase. They were not alarmed and felt able to manage his resolving condition should he relapse in the future. They also were made aware of 'Plan B' should things go awry. Everyone gets frightened.

One of our men, after a relatively settled period began to assault. We immediately met as a team to review what might be happening. Had his recent birthday reminded him of his lost life after nearly two decades in medium or low secure environments? Had his, partially responsive schizophrenia once again overtaken our seemingly feeble medication attempts? Was he, as an experienced patient, secreting his tablets? The staff had noticed his toilet being flushed on two occasions following his medication. We decided to crush and dissolve his clozapine, check the blood level and temporarily increase his benzodiazepine, but without involving him in the decision. His clozapine level came back and was consistent, if not slightly higher than they had been previously, confirming his self report of compliance. I apologised to him and ceased dissolving his tablets.

Later another concern about the risk of assault began to develop. Again, we sat with him as a team and outlined our concerns. We invited him to explore what might be happening. He remained steadfast, shrugged his shoulders and said "Don't know." We had been advised when he was transfered to us that he responded to clear and decisive direction, with attempts at physical escort only escalating into further violence. A third incident occurred. I invited him to the extra care area. He declined. I was now frightened.

It felt as if we were being held hostage by the advice we had been given at handover. He also reminded staff of another person who had assaulted them unexpectedly. There was a heightened sense that something was going to happen, that we should be doing something, and that someone was going to get hurt. We would then be asked to explain why we hadn't done anything. I wanted him transferred back to a medium secure unit but was aware I was reacting from fear. We knew a medium secure unit was unlikely to take him on the basis of what was happening. We also wondered about a short-term transfer to our Psychiatric Intensive Care Unit (PICU) but as they pointed out, what would they do differently that we couldn't with our own safe areas? We noted how our language changed. We talked about him 'bullying others', 'having the upper hand', of becoming 'the top dog' and that 'he was now in control' which seemed to add to our fear. Sitting with him however, you couldn't help but see a man, psychotic, struggling with experiences which he had previously communicated to us about others cutting, biting, assaulting and ripping his nose from his own face when he wasn't aware. We also knew as a team, for him, and for the other men, we needed to re-steady ourselves on this particular tightrope.

At the week's community meeting when activities for the day are discussed and decided individually, the issue of how best to help others who were struggling was raised. When he asked for his usual leave and this was declined, he asked why. We let him know it was because he had been hitting people. This enabled all of us to be aware we were responding to his change in circumstances. Those who had witnessed his most recent assault, watched this closely and nodded in agreement. Later, I asked him whether he had minded having these matters discussed in the community meeting. He hadn't minded at all. I just wanted to check.

This situation required gentle but confident discussion with the person rather than allowing language to heighten or divide the team, and for reflection on the planned response. When we became calmer, the person also had the opportunity to regain his composure. When we asked again how we could best help him and what had happened at his previous medium secure unit, he was able to say they did what we were doing. With our fear contained he was able to re-contain his own experiences.

A tricky thing fear. It is rapidly contagious and debilitating. But also understandable and manageable. It requires a united and committed team that can talk through the issues.

two

Once we felt safe …

"Treat people as if they were what they ought to be and you will help them become what they are capable of becoming."

Van Goethe

4

Who would have thought?

When I was young I was lucky enough to work for the Waipukurau Borough Council repairing roads and collecting rubbish.

Bob, the boss was probably in his 50s or 60s. He drove the council truck, an old green Bedford, to the various jobs. On this particular day he was drunk but seemed to slip the truck into gear in the same way he was slurring his speech.

We pulled up outside the hospital where the kerb of the footpath was broken. Bob got me to mix up the concrete while he managed to haul himself back into the cab and slumped into a deep sleep. I wasn't quite sure how to go about this. I was 15 and although I knew about 'boxing up', it wasn't easy to drive stakes in to keep the board in place, the gutter also being concrete. I placed the length of board along the gutter on its edge and tried to wedge it against the footpath edge. I poured the concrete in, mixed it a bit dry and hoped for the best. Even before I walked away I could see it starting to ooze. When we visited it the next day it had, but it did the job and people were able to walk on the footpath again. This is one of many bedtime stories I told our children and never really thought a lot else about it.

Maybe some 30 years later when we took our children back home to show them New Zealand, we were driving in Waipukurau. I was driving into town and suddenly pulled the van over to the side and said "Everybody out!" They all looked a bit bewildered, couldn't see anything of particular note that would warrant getting out, but hopped out anyway. I was so excited. I hurried them back and said "Look, there it is, the footpath I always told you about!" Rosie, our eldest, was delighted. She thought it was the highlight of the trip. Who would have thought something I had done at the age of 15, would have had such an impact some 30 odd years later!

Lee

Lee was in his late 20s. He had been in the mental health system from his teens. His clothes were filthy. He seldom wore underpants and his jeans were slung down low. His hair and beard were incredibly long, greasy and matted. Lee had not wanted to wash and wouldn't allow anyone else to wash him or his hair, even though he had been on the unit for some time. He was largely uncommunicative, his face hidden.

He came to me one day and asked how long would it take for him to get out of here. He wanted to set himself a goal. I was speechless and returned to the team wondering how to respond. We didn't want to appear hopeless or discouraging, but equally we didn't want to be unrealistic. We suggested perhaps six to 12 months, deliberately vague and non-committal as we were not expecting any changes as none had happened to date.

Within six weeks, Lee had changed. He allowed the staff to clean, shampoo, un-matt and cut his hair – an exercise which took some days. He shaved, changed his clothes, cut his nails and began to talk and smile. He wanted leave.

Initially we tried five minutes leave within the hospital grounds and he had to get himself a watch in order to get back on time. He agreed and with a smile, came back and said he had also bought himself a belt! Lee continued to do well, buying himself new clothes, and increasing his leave. Although there were the occasional hiccups, turned his life around to the extent he was able to progress to Fettle House, our open mixed rehabilitation unit.

I still bump into him and he always greets me with a great big smile and handshake. I am still not sure what made the difference. It may have been because one of the men who had been particularly disruptive was transferred off the unit. This enabled not only Lee, but a number of other people to come out of their rooms and begin to engage in the activity programme. It may have been because two of the other men had already started to move from Bowman to Fettle House. Maybe it was the result of seeing his peers leave that made the difference. We still don't know.

There was no change of medication and Lee's change remains as remarkable as Rosie's recollection of bedtime stories years earlier. Who would have thought?

When I first met Dean I wasn't able to stay in the same room with him for more than a couple of minutes. His conversation was so thought disordered I was unable to make any sense, or know where to begin let alone know how to proceed.

Dean was first admitted to hospital when he was 15. Despite multiple and high dose combinations of medications; none had had any effect. I didn't know what to do, so I decided I would just sit down and talk with him. I tried to get a sense of what he was trying to say through his thought disorder. I tried to paraphrase it then watched him to see whether I was anywhere near to what he wanted to say. It reminded me of many years ago when I studied psychology and we were given letters written by people with schizophrenia. Somehow these letters engaged me. I could see, rather than being 'schizophrenic', this was a person trying to communicate, albeit in a slightly different way. I didn't know how Dean and I began to talk but it seemed to be a similar sort of thing. Just trying to make sense of what he was saying somehow made a difference. Who would have thought?

I wouldn't have thought it possible

There are two other examples I want to add in to this section because prior to my arrival, and informed only by the great trickster, prejudice, I wouldn't have thought it was possible.

Like many units, we have a community meeting each morning. On Thursdays I attend to raise issues about the unit atmosphere and ask about any specific concerns. As you can imagine, most of the meetings are relatively mundane and related to house keeping.

However, I was genuinely surprised how thoughtful the men were about contentious issues and how conservative they were in their positions. Particularly to their views on drugs, alcohol and on violent and pornographic videos. We had quite an animated debate about these topics. The men recognised there was a need for balance although some things were just totally unacceptable. For example, the men were able to identify different individuals may require different consequences as a result, for example of drinking on leave. While we tried to treat everyone the same, there were also individual circumstances. Accordingly the unit didn't become split over what may have been regarded as unfairness. Again I'm not really sure how this developed and it certainly doesn't happen every week, but the fact it does happen is remarkable. We've included some examples of the community meetings in Appendix 1. Who would have thought?

Three men

The final example relates to three of our men who performed in a music gig at a Mental Health Forum in Plymouth in March 2010. I was aware of the informal support we as staff members offer each other, and how this stands in contrast to the individual men on the unit who seemingly share little other than a light for their cigarettes.

Lee who had moved on to Fettle House, Rehabilitation Unit, Zach and Tom who had come to us having accumulated over 100 pages of police incidents, all got together under the enthusiasm and commitment of Adrian and Nigel. Together they formed a band and regularly rehearsed. Three individuals with three quite different backgrounds, and despite Adrian having the flu, Lee having pneumonia and Zach possibly relapsing in the week before the gig, all managed to get to Plymouth, perform, get photographed and return without incident. Who would have thought?

It seems important that the quotation at the start of this chapter is repeated:

"Treat people as if they were what they ought to be and you will help them to become what they are capable of being."

Says it all really doesn't it?

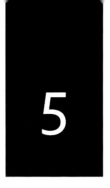

5 Feeling safe

"If only there were evil people insidiously committing evil deeds and it were necessary to separate them from the rest of us and destroy them. But the line dividing good and evil will cut through the heart of every human being and who is willing to destroy a piece of his own heart."

Solzhenitsyn

Initial Impressions from a novice

For a long time I wasn't sure how the team, in particular Iain and Will, had been able to create a feeling of safety amidst a warm, homelike atmosphere. I went to London with them to a Security in Forensic Settings Conference. These men were hilarious, tears of laughter were streaming down my face. Gifted clinicians, great men who have that rare ability to be themselves and to form easy relationships with a wide range of people.

We agreed it was quite difficult to write this section because what they had been able to do was to create a system of unobtrusive safety mechanisms.

I then began to think about my arrival at Bowman on the first and subsequent days. There is no obvious signage or indication to suggest I was entering a low secure unit. I pressed the intercom button outside the door, somebody came and welcomed me into the air lock, provided me with a security alarm, showed me how to use it and walked with me to the office.

The unit has a lovely garden area thanks to a regular and generous donation from Mrs Banham. There is a landscaped area with varying foliage, summer seating and a small allotment carefully attended to by our occupational therapist (OT), Mark. Staff later pointed out the fence (which I hadn't really noticed as it seemed to blend into the background), was made of anti-climbing mesh. We were going to have a routine review of our service and we asked a couple of the men to help us shift the garden shed. It was close to the wall of an adjacent building and there was the possibility of someone being able to climb onto the roof and abscond. I hadn't noticed that either. Nor had I noticed the anti-rolling material on the guttering. We readily passed the review, Iain having pitched the security level to meet the standard for a medium secure setting.

One recommendation from this review suggested we put in an additional 16 CCTV cameras. It seemed a bit excessive as things seemed to be going okay, but again it turned out to be particularly helpful in an unexpected way.

When someone reported bullying, a staff member was hit, and a serious allegation of impropriety was made by one of the men against three of our staff members, CCTV footage was invaluable. We were able to sit with each of the men and show them what had actually happened. The bullying was confronted, the assault to the staff member led to a police intervention and the allegation which could have led to the immediate suspension and termination of employment was seen for what it actually was, a malicious complaint in retaliation to a grievance. CCTV also enabled confirmation of a genuine complaint. Matters were dealt with swiftly by talking rather than tackling.

Ian our new psychologist (whose clear potential at interview was confirmed within a very short period of time) commented, that in contrast to previous units where he had worked, there was a sense of wanting to manage potentially volatile situations differently on Bowman Unit. Based on his observations in previous clinical settings Ian described how the use of restraint can impact on a unit's culture. He explained how the process of restraint can lead to a sense of camaraderie between the staff who have been through such an acutely challenging situation together. While this allows staff to be mutually supportive, Ian commented it is important the desire to maintain the sense of camaraderie doesn't lead to restraint being used as anything less than a last resort.

I was also impressed by the daily handover. In particular, how each staff member was invited, or in fact required to, write on the handover form for each shift. How each morning, events, observations and concerns were relayed. I had vaguely heard about piecing together seemingly isolated scraps of information which then suddenly made sense but hadn't really experienced it before.

We were in a handover meeting and I ventured to say that I had wondered whether or not Mr A had looked at my groin. Somehow it had made me feel uncomfortable. I felt somewhat embarrassed to mention it, but also felt it might be important. Karen also made an observation as did another staff member, and then yet another recalled background information relating to Mr A - sexuality and violence. All of a sudden it clicked. We recognised Mr A might be beginning to become unwell and assaultative again. These observations seemingly isolated and unrelated, were early warnings of something building up. We won't know for sure whether we were able to avert a possible attack, but being able to talk about our concerns was important.

My immediate predecessor, Russell, contributed enormously to the unit. I felt Russell's event planning forms were reassuring. With an electronically available template, Russell set up a format in which the specific risks for each individual were spelt out. Details of any escorted and unescorted leave under Section 17 including time periods, specific locations and distances from the hospital and/or the index offence, and the purposes for each leave including where relevant, the number and gender of escorts per trip, were indicated. Those who were vulnerable were reminded with each leave that this was an opportunity for them to demonstrate to themselves as well as to us what they were now capable of achieving. It just felt safer.

Similarly and again thanks to Russell's initiative the HCR-20 (a tool used to think about a person's risk) was available for each patient with specific sections being delegated to different members of the team according to their professional discipline. John and Bernie from the community forensic team taught us well, highlighting a structured approach actually did provide a useful function and although we completed them a little superficially to start with, they did end up being very useful reminders of the extent of the risk. With our new psychologist on board we have a very robust focus on specific scenarios and their management.

Like many small and rural communities, people know one another. Will and Tim had been friends at school. Will was now a staff nurse on a low secure unit; Tim had an acquired brain injury and was being referred to our unit. We needed to talk about it.

Will interestingly made the same comment Tim made when we later discussed it with him, "It feels weird." Will went on to reflect about the experiences they had together growing up, and how life becomes serious, never knowing quite what is going to happen next. He understood the dilemmas and potential issues and as we all agreed, Will couldn't be Tim's primary nurse. Will also saw the value of going up and meeting Tim while he was on the psychiatric intensive care unit, partly in order to catch up as they hadn't seen each other for years, and partly to talk through some of the issues.

We let Tim know we were coming, and interestingly he had shaven and got dressed up. It was important for him. Will outlined issues that were significant for him and explained that at times he may need to direct Tim but he wouldn't be responsible for him on a primary basis. We had already agreed, as a team, it would be somebody else who would take Tim down to the unit to show him around, somebody else would administer his depot and that he would arrive on a day when Will wasn't on duty. Together they were able to be open, honest and direct, be clear about things and to acknowledge, sadly, their relationship had changed for ever. Interestingly, Tim himself, was able to recognise it would take some time to come to terms with meeting up and now having a different relationship with his friend. He could also see there were advantages as he knew there were good people on the unit, namely Michaela who he had worked with previously, and now Will.

This is Will's account:

Will and Tim

If you think the world is a small place try living in Cornwall! Having dished out 'harmless ridicules' to another member staff, who had recently been placed in the very awkward position of nursing a former acquaintance, I too soon found myself to have been placed in this difficult position. I had known Tim and had gone to school with him from the age of 13 to 16. I had also attended Cornwall College with Tim after leaving school. We both shared similar interests and had the same group of friends. We had lost contact with one another, as people do with certain friends, after I left our home town at the age of 19.

I had some concerns that Tim would divulge personal information about my past, but at the same time felt he would respect my professional standing on the unit, which has been the case to date.

I had known Tim had been admitted to another unit within the Trust and a subsequent referral had been made to Bowman Unit. I fed back to members of the team that Tim had been a friend of mine and this could pose an issue for both of us if he were to be offered a placement on Bowman. A recent assessment had been carried out and Tim had provisionally been offered the opportunity to be transferred into the care of the

Bowman Team. Prior to any formal decision being made it felt important Tim and I met each other. I found this, as I am sure Tim did, a very odd and surreal situation to have been placed in, and how the circumstances around our relationship had changed. From the outset I had felt it important, for myself and Tim, to take 'a back seat' in regards to planning Tim's programme of care. I think it has been of benefit for Tim to have an old acquaintance on the unit and I hope it has been a positive experience for him also.

I feel both Tim and I have on occasion struggled with professional boundaries, but have been able to overcome this due to our past relationship and have on numerous occasions been able to normalise certain situations. I feel Tim and I have had a mutual understanding and trust from the outset and that this has been advantageous in times of crisis. I think this 'quirk of fate' highlights how any of us could, at any time, be affected by mental illness and how this impacts on everyday life. Tim and I have discussed how it could have easily been me in his position and him in the role of the clinician. This has enabled us to reflect and has aided us throughout, giving us both mutual empathy and understanding instead of a more formal relationship.

Similarly, Jess knew one of our other men when they

were at school together. Dan said they used to hang around the arcade together and were boyfriend and girlfriend for a couple of weeks, as you do at that age, but it was a long time ago. Even so, it was important for us to be able to talk it through with Jess and the team in order to clarify any hesitations Jess may have. When we asked Jess, she thought about it for a while and wrote the following.

Jess and Dan

Cornwall is often described as 'one big village', meaning everyone knows everyone. So it didn't really come as a surprise when we received a referral for a guy called Dan, who I had had a brief relationship with when I was approximately 14 years old. Initially I was filled with dread and very anxious about his proposed admission. I informed the rest of the team about our history and was expectedly met with a lot of harmless ridicule, but also with a lot of support. My biggest fear was he would/could blackmail me by divulging information from our past to the other patients or staff.

The first shift I worked after Dan's admission I remember feeling very anxious, I reluctantly introduced myself, asked if he remembered me (which he did) and was honest about how I was feeling anxious about working with him. I asked how he felt about being on the same unit I worked on. Fortunately he didn't have a problem with me working there and he has always been totally respectful of me as a member of staff and of our history.

Again it was the opportunity to be able to identify potential risk, to talk about it openly and to clearly and confidently put it to rest. I think that about says it. Bowman has a very strong emphasis on relational security. It is this which is unobtrusive.

From a security viewpoint

As the Charge Nurse and Security Lead for Bowman Unit when John asked for a contribution to this work on the area of security, a tidal wave of nausea swept through my soul. This is clearly not a topic easily delivered without including the usual clinical standards, fully risk assessed by three external review teams' data. "Fences, cameras, searches, alarms, airlocks, observation, prohibition, testing, the minor point of respectful and genuine engagement, heights, widths, lengths, gaps, ligatures, leaves etc etc etc." Seeing my reaction, John kindly reframed the question, and asked me to consider honestly how Bowman had evolved so far (and continues to) mostly safely. The new challenge now becomes how to avoid the well documented terminology.

I think it would be fair to state that around the country, there are low secures that resemble medium secures, medium secure units that resemble youth hostels and youth hostels that resemble high secures. Standards allow some national commonality, but the key issue is to ensure the delivery matches the character of specific counties. In the early days, we were clearly weaker in some areas of safety. What was lacking in experience however was balanced by emphasis on engagement driven by a 'whole life principle'. This has now been augmented by the 'Camilla System' which is described below. While we continue to evolve, it remains a finely balanced eco system.

Here's the low secure conundrum. We would like you to create a 14-bedded unit, from a building designed for another purpose. Inhabit it with a group of system-battered gentlemen who will be held against their will, who will likely have danced on the wrong side of the law and enable them to take the final step from a secure setting into a welcoming community. We would like this unit to mirror the likely living setting of the community, but without blind spots, ligature points or easily movable furniture.

We hope and expect you to form genuine relationships and engage in therapeutic and educational activities with the men on the unit, but only after you search, drug-screen and lock both doors behind them. Encourage and enhance daily living skills but without instant access to the necessary sharp utensils required for the task. We also want to take positive risks and smoothly integrate our inhabitants into the community without attracting the great eye of 'SAURON'. Here goes!

For those of you who watch 'Doc Martin' or are Cornish you may have heard the phrase "He's gone Bodmin."

Bodmin is a small town and historically housed a large county asylum and jail. Bodmin Hospital sits on the outskirts of the town. The town inhabitants and local communities have a special relationship with the hospital. It is likely if you are not related to someone who works in the hospital you will almost certainly know someone who works there, or indeed has been there as a patient. While this proximity may bring issues including privacy, there is also a sense of genuine acceptance of mental ill health in Bodmin, which does not naturally occur without intensive community education. This hand in hand with a huge geographical land mass, a low socio-economic status and fickle transport system, some how make Section 17 leave in this area of the country more readily accepted. There will be few areas of the country that have 'the local garage' as a defined part of Section 17 leave or a local garage which rings the hospital reception rather than the local police to highlight a potential incident!

We have a beautifully designed garden on Bowman, which needed royal approval and a grand opening by HRH the Duches of Cornwall, Camilla Parker Bowles. While not naive enough to think Camilla would pitch up in a Bodmin cab, drink tea, pull the curtain on the plaque and be on her royal way, the following normally unseen activity enhanced the concept of how low secure safety should work.

The pre-arrival tasks of the royal visit included a full screening of all people who would be in the vicinity of the garden on the arranged day, including their criminal and political beliefs. Only a pre-ordained list of people would have direct access to the Duchess of Cornwall. An assessment of the garden, access and egress, two bomb sweeps, and the identification of a designated safe area were all made. Multiple meetings with a royal protection officer (whose genuine name was Bond!) to discuss routes, timetables for all plus a list of dos and don'ts was undertaken.

On the day Camilla arrived, she waved and walked down the corridor to meet the pre-arranged people. A friendly German psychiatrist, oblivious to the preparation, had joined the dignitary queue and was discretely removed by a security officer. To an onlooker, Camilla may have looked unprotected and at risk in the garden. However, she was standing in a garden with a

'3.5m single wield mesh fence with a 45 degree inward angle with external fence posts and no obvious footholds'. Although not obvious, the safety of Camilla and her escorts had been carefully considered and none of the 'suited, earpiece-wearing security guy's' were visible. If something had happened most eventualities had been thought through.

This unobtrusive 'Camilla System' is replicated in Bowman. Security is in the background, not obvious and doesn't intrude upon the overall philosophy, culture or feel of the unit. Everyone present has a clear role. Everyone that needs information has the right information, and monitoring is specific to individuals. If anything goes wrong, immediate contingencies are in place. People not used to the environment need direction and care. That same environment needs to be clear of potential hazards. The task is focused in order to create a safe but home-like environment. As part of these guidelines there is an overarching philosophy that anyone who visits, lives or works should not have to go about their daily business feeling frightened or at risk. The words communally and inclusivity have to be embraced in a genuine manner.

In addition to the 'Camilla System' we use the daily handover with staff, the daily community meeting with the guys and the larger weekly community meeting where the consultant attends, to review any breaches in safety. These allow discussions to be genuinely opened up and debated. The whole unit can contribute to risk awareness and management. Although appearing insignificant, a recent concern whereby a couple of clients were using up to 16 sachets of sugar each for breakfast was raised. 'Not a security issue' I hear you shout! However, our concern was that by attempting to control sugar intake, we may inadvertently create a sub-culture with a 'black market' which could lead to more vulnerable clients exchanging sugar for cigarettes, money, property. This could in turn lead swiftly to debt, bullying, fear, disengagement and subsequent failure to reach their 'potential' in this environment. This was discussed at the community meeting and resolved.

Finally, I recently flew into San Francisco from New Zealand. I had to check in one hour earlier than usual, all my bags were emptied, shoes and socks removed, body scanned, fingers printed and eyes photographed. Although inconvenient, I felt some how reassured. Two days later, I boarded a plane to London. On this occasion all I had to do was to show my passport and go through a metal detector. In comparison I felt strangely under searched and unsafe. What this made me aware of was how quickly a level of safety became acceptable and crucially when I had been through both procedures and was on board I was treated kindly and respectfully with attention to my comfort, and choices of drinks, food and movies. Security can be matched to the individual and his particular risks.

Security doesn't have to get in the way of a personal service.

The team has been able to create a secure base from which we can explore and become adventurous in our rehabilitation efforts. We are happy to share our physical and procedural policies, but I think what makes the difference is an unspoken emphasis on what is called relational security. It is perhaps appropriate the next chapter is about our most valuable resource, our staff.

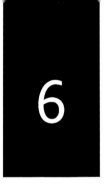

6

Interesting People

"For beautiful eyes look for the good in others, for beautiful lips, speak only words of kindness, and for poise, walk with the knowledge that you are never alone."

Audrey Hepburn

I'm still not quite sure whether to include a chapter on staffing or more particularly to name specific individuals. Naming some and not others may lead to the mistaken belief others are not as noteworthy. That's not true. I think that's why we decided to call this chapter 'Interesting People'. The other reason not everybody is mentioned is because what we have tried to do is capture those people who seem to represent individual characters which are present in every team, or for some reason we just happened to notice at the time. All of us are important and all of our names are at the back. Karen put it this way. "Within all walks of life there are people who stand out at either end of the scale. There are also all those people – in most cases the majority – who simply get on with things and without whom things would fail miserably."

Joyce is from the north. She is small, at least in size, maybe in her 50s, with white hair and lives in a caravan looking after her husband who is poorly. She has a lovely gentle style in the community meeting, not letting the men get away with inactivity, but also being able to coax and encourage them into signing up for at least something each day. She described how in a previous job in another county she had persisted in making the effort trying to find a Jewish connection for one of her patients.

Joyce

When I was working on a psychiatric intensive care unit, I had a patient who was an Orthodox Jewish gentleman.

One Saturday morning I went into work to find he could not celebrate Shabbat as he did not have the unleven bread or grape juice. I asked him if there was anywhere we could get these for him. He said if I went to see the Rabbi at his synagogue the Rabbi's wife would provide these for me. When I arrived at the synagogue I had to wait outside until someone came to ask if they would get the Rabbi to come outside to speak to me. Unfortunately the Rabbi had gone on holiday that weekend but a lady asked who I had come for. Not breaking patient confidentiality I explained I worked in a hospital and needed this food for a patient. The lady I spoke to said her cousin was in hospital (she actually named the hospital and the unit I worked on and even named my patient). She asked me to go to her house and said she would give me the food that was needed. I knew my patient would appreciate this and how it would make him feel better not only spiritually but mentally as well.

It was Joyce being Joyce - interested concerned and wanting to do her bit whatever it took.

Elizabeth had come up with an idea at the community meeting. I asked her about it afterwards. She said, she had been at home over the weekend, it was wet and miserable, and she wondered what she should do to fill in time and cheer herself up. She looked in the 'What's On' section of the paper and saw various Christmas shopping trips, car boot sales, fetes and Christmas Fayres, Par Market, Trelawney Garden Centre, the festive Christmas lights at Mousehole, evening shopping and trips to neighbouring towns. Rather than sitting at home, she went out and about. She then made the connection. If that's something I enjoy, maybe the men would as well. They did.

Marianne, our first psychologist, provided detailed, comprehensive and evidence based reports. More importantly she also modelled to the remainder of us the value of sitting and talking to people. Staff often commented when they saw one of the men coming out from one of her sessions with a big smile, 'What did you do, what did you say?' She also stuck with and was finally able to ensure reflective practice actually started.

Vanessa is extraordinarily gifted. She is gentle but not in that woolly, sickening way so well parodied on television. From experience, she gave us enough information to make us curious and enabled us to reconnect with a person who we may have inadvertently and momentarily lost as we became blinded by behaviour or illness.

Michaela is remarkable in practising what she preaches. She recognised reflective practice was not to everyone's taste and an individualised approach was just as important for staff as it was for our men.

Karen was quiet, small and seemed to sit in the background. However she got on with it - quick, quiet, efficient and effective. She was our new social worker. It transpired she was a mother at the age of 16 and now had four children. Remarkably she also runs competitively. Sadly she left, but was replaced by Annette. Wow! Within a short period of time her experience and background in domestic violence and child protection was evident. 'New blood' in an organisation makes such a difference.

Catch was cheeky with her Glaswegian accent. You could tease her and she would laugh. I asked her to make the doctor a cup of tea once and I got the reply you might expect! She was the same with the men as she was with us. With her cheeky, delightful grin she would say to Tony "You proper make me sick Tony" engaging and encouraging him to shower. He would take this on board as it was said with kindness and a genuine regard for him as a person who she cared about. People loved her. This was posted by a staff member: "Due to the fact we are not having a posh Christmas Party, an invite is going out to all staff to celebrate Christmas. Also I ain't being funny, but Catriona 'Princess' Canning is leaving the Bowman Team like in December so we thought it would be a good idea to give her 'like' a leaving party to remember, which will make her think 'like' that we are going to miss her 'like' and that she is 'proper lush'." She also had the rare ability to be open, honest and direct with men. Here's a lovely example of her work:

Catch

In anticipation of not being discharged from the act, Tom was a large and powerfully built man who presented as an intimidating person as he paced around the unit waiting for the hearing to commence. Rather than waiting, Catch could see the potential and took the initiative. She sat down with Tom and acknowledged he was stressed and outlined with him those reasons that were making him as unsettled as he had become. She began to explore rather than accept his first reply in relation to his abnormal experiences and the side effects to medication -

"I understand how you feel about it, but I see things differently and agree to disagree." Catch then used examples Tom himself had used and paraphrased these back to him – "You've told me how you've been hearing voices and seeing shadows. I can't imagine what that's like, it must be horrible. I just see myself and others here as normal people." Catch then went on to actually describe what was going on and said to Tom he could come across as scary and that she didn't like it when people were scared. "I want to be as honest as I can" and asked Tom how we could help if he got bad news and wasn't discharged from the Tribunal. Having had the opportunity to speak, be listened to and understood and to have an open, honest and direct discussion around the concerns identified, of assault or absconsion, Tom was able to reply on his own initiative suggesting maybe he could go outside in the garden afterwards. Tom was reassured it must be a real struggle for him without the use of drugs and alcohol, wanting to leave all the time and yet being locked up against his will.

Catch is in her 20s, Michaela in her 40s and Angela, the Consultant on Fettle House, rehabilitation unit in her 70s. They all have that rare skill; neither confrontational nor defiant, neither pleading nor wishful, but rather a matter of fact expectation, clearly, gently and warmly articulated. It enables Angela, with at least one artificial hip, to hobble into the bedroom and get the men up for their morning meeting! They get up because people know she is genuine, warm and committed to their well being. For those of us who are not blessed with these qualities, we could watch and try to model what they did naturally.

Will demonstrated this recently. Phil had taken Paul out for a ride and Paul with his characteristic black humour and wish to shock people, made some comment about cutting his throat with the folded £10 note he had in his hand. Phil correctly relayed this to the team. Paul wanted to put in a complaint as to how unfair it was, how he was just joking and how he always ended up on each unit longer than anyone else. Will replied "No that's not the case" and kept returning Paul to the actual reality "No, that's a separate issue", "No, Phil was doing his job," "No, that's not correct."

Phil is a Geordie. Rough and ready, completely bald, with a tooth or two missing and maybe in his late 40s. He has seen quite a bit of life and what a big hearted, generous man. Engaging and always happy to help out with a big warm grin that straight away puts you at ease. Just being himself without judging is Phil's gift.

Adrian and Ian made significant musical contributions. Adrian dragged himself into work for the final rehearsal before the guys' musical gig in Plymouth, despite looking dreadful with winter flu.

Matt took me under his wing and looked after me on the Personal Safety Training Course. I was impressed by Godwin's gentle presence, stepping in between Catch and one of the men who was becoming agitated. Godwin was one of the regular men from the bank staff who was sought after by a number of the units, as were Vicky and Perry. Thanks Alice.

It's interesting to think about the men as a group as although there are possibly more female staff, the men provide an important balance on the unit. Although there is an easy going banter, there remains a mutual and professional respect for each other as colleagues without sexual tension or rivalry. That Michaela is female, is the unit manager who developed and fostered the philosophy of the unit, and I am male, the consultant on the unit is of note as the unit began to settle.

Are there downsides to staffing?

Yes. At first I didn't want to have this section. I was tempted to present just the 'good'. It was Vanessa who pointed out how it may have been too uncomfortable for one of our men to explore his 'bad' side, presenting himself instead as 'the model patient'. It is uncomfortable to mention the 'bad side' of our staffing, dishonest and unhelpful. I was encouraged by my wife to read this extraordinary quotation from a novel she was reading at the time "... the belligerent apathy of those who turn their job into a platform for obstructing the life of others." What a brilliant distillation of ideas and imagery! To be honest, I haven't seen a lot of this on our unit but have previously seen it. I think that's why the quote jumped out at me, for it succinctly characterised a small section of the various workforces I had been in over the years. That it doesn't just occur in mental health suggests it is a universal observation.

Michaela deliberately never identified to me any staff with whom she had particular difficulties. I asked her about this once and she said firstly, she had spent quite a bit of time carefully selecting the team which she had built up with those attributes she felt were important. So while lots of the staff had come from different backgrounds, she saw this as important as it brought a mixture of experiences and views. It also enabled Michaela to recognise people had their own personal interests which they could bring to share with the men on the unit; music, photography, gardening, cycling and now with the arrival of Ian, even parachuting! From the start she saw very much the importance of getting and keeping the staff that worked with us. We have a 5% turnover per year which provides an all important continuity and secure base.

For those Michaela has had difficulty with, usually their manner or approach, she described managing them by being open, honest and direct. She would sit down in supervision, ask whether they were happy on the unit and if not, in what way could she help them get to where they might want to be? I thought this was respectful and an acknowledgement, that the slow pace of a rehabilitation and recovery focused low secure unit might not suit everyone.

Michaela was able to focus on the task rather than the person. People appreciate the honesty she has. She continues to see strengths in people and gives them opportunities while being able to stay in the background and allow them to take on their new role. Sometimes it requires careful attention to the rostering of which staff are on duty with each other. It includes not being afraid of carefully trying, matching and if need be, changing staff rosters in order to prevent splits and to promote a cohesion. She is a natural leader.

There were two Beckys on our unit, both were lovely. It seemed they were very talented and important members of our team who contributed enormously and without whom we couldn't function. I wasn't surprised to later find Becky had a degree in psychology and was looking forward to using her skill with supervision from our new psychologist. Our other Becky was our unit secretary and like all unit secretaries invaluable. Doing all those little things without fuss and enabling the smooth running of the unit. I wanted her to write a section on her experiences as a unit secretary but she giggled and said she'd be fine but would put her bit in the book meeting.

Michaela recognised Sarah's energy and enthusiasm,

and offered her a six month opportunity of Acting Social Inclusion Officer. Paul had been seconded elsewhere for a period of time. She bounded into the job as you can tell from this e-mail:

Sarah

Hi Michaela and John

Just let you know I held the meeting, it was a very good one! Finished at five! We all talked for three hours!!! Before I did anything about it thought I'd run it by you both first, (I will Friday if you both think its ok and I will look into it all further and arrange)

Anyway if it's ok with you I have a lady from C.V who's a service user and has another support carer with her and would love to bake somewhere different..., after chats it could every week :) and I said could it just be just cake and sweet things so as not to clash with Mark's shared lunch. Also I got the name of a farm who may take some of the men for work experience, proper work :) also a place with animals people can feed etc ;) also contact details who's giving out funding for a self empowerment group, which sounds great. And if possible, I was thinking it could be a social fund for the men on the unit and they can run it. I have to speak to them as it's a community thing and see where we stand as we are a locked unit. They gave one group three grand :) Also found some friends!!!! (not for me) but for the men on the unit, Re-think have people who offer friendship as I asked about this the other day as poor old Mr A said to me once, all he wants is a friend. I had an idea while we sat there what's your take is on it? If I can get the local snooker hall in town to give us the place for the afternoon or something, even better as a regular slot and get the 'friends' and our men having snooker matches off the unit, also would be poss. to get men to meet in the nearest coffee shop and have a coffee chat group to would be good?? Well I'm over-loaded :)

See you Friday, Sarah xxx

With time, Sarah also began to see her role was not just including the men in finding and supporting them in opportunities and experiences they had never had before, but also included supporting those organisations that were accepting our men.

Siobhan was also interesting. At first I hadn't noticed her ability. It wasn't perhaps until Catch left that I watched her clearly and decisively handle a crisis on the unit and saw immediately why she deserved her place as the lead staff nurse on her shift. Sarah was very clear in her views and as I began to get to know her, she told me she had come from a high secure adolescent unit. She was an important member of the team who was able to challenge colleagues including myself to prevent 'group think' and did so when we were slowly and gradually moving Paul to Fettle House, rehabilitation unit.

We love the UK, love the people, the accents, and the humour! While the work is at times hard, the team is remarkable: thoughtful, experienced, decisive and funny. Finally, I would like to finish by quoting Lord Layard who was director of the Wellbeing Programme of the LSE Centre for Economic Performance. He wrote this commentary in The Guardian on July 14, 2007, just over three years ago as a letter to the incoming Secretaries of State advising them to be careful of "change for change sake" and of restructuring. As I re-read this, you can't help but think that once again it remains timely.

He starts of by saying:

> "You have a wonderful opportunity to improve public services. No doubt you have reflected on the efforts of the last 20 years; but here, if you are interested, are a few thoughts. On my reading the lesson is this: high morale and good policy should be the priority and major reorganisations a last resort.
>
> Reorganisation is much less important than some think. In fact, many different organisational structures can be made to work equally well. What can not work is constant reorganisation, where nobody understands what is happening, institutional memory is lost and everybody

worries about their future rather than the job in hand ...

Your main priority must be the morale of your service, since without it we can not deliver for the public. This means telling staff clearly what is wanted and using public spirit as the source of motivation: it is your greatest treasure. Never slag off the team and monitor morale meticulously.

The task is not to devise clever incentive schemes which assume that no one will do their job properly unless they are paid extra every time they do so. The cheap instruments for promoting quality and spreading good practice are clear objectives, good benchmarking, lifelong training, supportive management, rigorous inspection and objective funding.

Objectives can be extremely useful, even if achieving them has no effect on pay. Pay must be sufficient to attract the right people into the right responsibility. Once a person is in a post, their dominant aim must be to gain the respect of superiors and colleagues.

To promote good team work, we do not need individual performance related pay. It reduces co-operation between colleagues and it discourages as much as it encourages. So much needs doing to improve services people get and high morale is the key".

Quite an interesting and thoughtful read that I suspect remains as relevant today as it did three years ago.

three

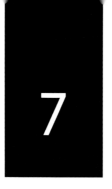

7 Positive risk taking

When I first worked in Cornwall some five years ago, one of the things that struck me was how risk averse public sector psychiatrists seemed to be, certainly in comparison with Australasia. People were in hospital for longer periods of time than I was used to. The Australasians appear to take a more pragmatic approach to risk than our UK counterparts.

When I arrived on the low secure unit and began to meet the men I realised, I had in Australia, managed a not dis-similar population in the community. That is, they appeared relatively settled, despite long histories. Perhaps naively, and perhaps denying risk as a defence, I decided to do it differently.

It seemed the safest position was to acknowledge the difficulties and sit safely with everyone locked up. However, there was also the expectation the men would be on the unit for up to two years, and so some forward planning was needed to enable them to move on. Feeling out of my depth and inexperienced, I went to various forums on low secure environments, all of which tended to focus and emphasise risk - risk assessment, risk management, separating risk from safety etc etc.

Certainly some tools have been quite useful and in particular those such as the HCR-20 and RSVP (tools used to think about a person's risk) which serve to bring together disparate bits of information and remind the team caution is required. Somewhere along the line, careful risk is required.

With this in mind, we took some risks.

Paul had been in the system for over 25 years. He seemed content to stretch out on the outdoor lounge furniture, or wander through the unit in his T-shirt, track pants and sandals. He related well to the staff, being a warm and jovial person with an engaging smile and wicked sense of humour. Concerns were expressed about the possibility of him moving to Fettle House, the open rehabilitation unit. Various meetings with Fettle, the community forensic team and his mum ensued. We agreed to try, over a six month period, to gradually and supportively enable the transfer. As we discussed earlier in the book, symptoms that had previously appeared quiescent began to re-emerge. Correctly these were recorded and presented for consideration. The illustrative point we wish to make on this occasion is again not new, but worth making all the same.

Potentially there could have been a split in the team with one group increasingly emphasising risk while the other diminishing it. We could have become distracted by egos or by different and previous clinical experiences. Each position also needed to be understood. In order for Paul to move forward, there had to be a united position which would enable the supportive process to come into play. We were reminded of the phenomenon known as 'group think'.

From memory, the phenomenon of group think arose out of the Cuban missile crisis or the failed Apollo space mission. It is when a group continues with an idea, seemingly swept up with the seduction of everyone agreeing but in so doing, fails to see the cracks. The suggestion for avoiding this phenomenon also forms an interesting way to think about risk. The processes in group think are: 1) the illusion of invulnerability where members ignore obvious danger, take extreme risk, and are overly enthusiastic. 2) Collective rationalisation where members discredit and explain away warnings and ignore the ethical implications of their decision. 3) Excessive stereotyping and the pressure for conforming, where the group creates negative stereotypes and challenges those who express arguments against the group, seeing opposition not as offering a unique perspective, but as disloyalty. As a result, members withhold their dissenting views and counter-arguments and believe falsely, that everyone agrees with the group's decision. Silence is seen as consent with some members assuming the role of protecting the group from adverse information which might threaten group complacency. Recognising these processes and dealing with the issues ensures we were unified over Paul's transfer. He was successfully transferred down to Fettle House, rehabiliation unit. A huge achievement for him.

Owen was a young man who was on our unit and appeared the 'model patient'. He was insightful, took his medication and managed his escorted and unescorted leave - all a little too good to be true. While he had only been on our unit for a relatively short period of time, five or six months, it was difficult to know how to clarify his idealised presentation without testing it in the community. Aware alcohol had previously been a problem, we wondered whether escorted visits to a pub would help Owen learn to socialise over a soft drink and a meal. We explored with him the thoughts, urges or feelings that might tempt him back into alcohol. We thought it was a reasonable plan. This is an account of what happened and is described by Adrian, who accompanied Owen for the leave.

Owen

There were obvious risks taking Owen to a local club, especially with his history, but, after a long period of settled behaviour we felt, if we tried to safeguard against every foreseeable outcome, we could reward his good behaviour and make an assessment of how he might behave in the community.

Myself (Healthcare Assistant), John (Psychiatrist) and Owen sat down and tried to establish what could go wrong. It was explained to Owen he would not be able to drink any alcohol and line of sight observations would be maintained at all times excluding the toilet cubicle (phew – could've been embarrassing!). It was also explained to Owen that at the first sign of any trouble, on my prompt, we were to return immediately to the vehicle. If Owen did not comply with this it would become a police matter. He was fine with all of this and assured us there would be no problems. Owen behaved impeccably the whole time, but a couple of issues arose that we just could not see coming.

The first of these was when we were outside the nightclub having a cigarette. A taxi pulled up and out fell three scantily clad Britney look-alikes – hubba hubba!! Unfortunately one of them was a friend of Owen and blurted out his offence to her mates in front of a queue of about 30 party goers!! We removed ourselves discreetly from the situation and slunk back into the club.

Another issue that arose was that somebody actually recognised Owen in the club and was aware of his offence even though we were some 30 miles away from Owen's home town. How would people in his home town react when they were aware he was out clubbing?

Little did I know, Owen was a bit of a babe magnet. A little while later he began dancing with an attractive young lady. I must admit I became a little self conscious at this point being 20 years older than most people in the club and having to maintain line of sight observations while their bodies gyrated provocatively against one anothers. I melted into the shadows when they began to kiss passionately on the dance floor. I must have looked quite a pervert stood there apparently leering from the corner! We left the club, grabbed a kebab and headed for home. As well as the food in our bellies that night I was left with plenty of food for thought..."

The reason for raising this incident in this section is to describe the feedback we received the next day from three concerned community forensic team members who each rang me separately. It was useful and supportive rather than critical and damning. They had sought clarification and made some useful suggestions about what now seems obvious. Raising a log number with the local police, ensuring there were no victim issues and ensuring the community forensic team were involved, could have contributed an added perspective prior to implementing the plan. However, what was important was as a result of this event, and the helpful way in which the feedback occurred, an opportunity was created by which Bowman, the community forensic team and (as it transpired) Fettle House, rehabiliation unit could begin to re-think about alcohol issues in the management of our specific populations. This work, which now includes the team from the drug and alcohol arm of the service, is ongoing.

Mr A was a young man who appeared to be relatively settled. He seemed to transfer without difficulty to Fettle House. He readily and eagerly participated and contributed in their activities programme. Mr A reported he wanted to stay on Fettle for a further three months as he recognised he still had work to do. He was clear he would be compliant with medication, having previously been readmitted after stopping his medication. He acknowledged he had an illness but these symptoms were now in abeyance. I felt he no longer met criteria for detention under the Mental Health Act. As you might guess, things did not work out quite as nicely as expected.

Fortunately his relapse was quickly identified from his early warning signs. As he had only recently been discharged seven weeks earlier, the sensible thing to do seemed to be just to re-admit him to Bowman Unit. Mr A returned and interestingly it took five to six months to stabilise him, despite initially putting him back on the medication which helped last time.

The temptation would have been to sit and not to consider discharge again, or at least not for a very long time. Taking a risk however, has afforded Mr A and us the opportunity of learning and understanding under what circumstances the plan fell down and how things might be done differently. It also became an opportunity for Bowman and Fettle to share and jointly develop a care pathway for this man. A pathway which has continued for our other men.

Risk taking also comes in other guises. It might have been tempting to adhere to the original admission criteria for an low secure unit. However, as our confidence grew, we began to carve out our own identity. We began to offer admissions to people who ordinarily may not have met low secure unit criteria but who may benefit from what Bowman had to offer.

One man who may not have met our initial admission criteria was Tim who had an acquired brain injury. We discussed as a team whether we might have something to offer. It might be that all we would be able to do is confirm that, sadly, Tim was unlikely to get better. We may also be able to provide relief for an exhausted community team and acute unit. Both goals would be important.

I am also reminded of Tom who came to us with 86 police incidents mainly for petty crime. He had been a major absconding risk from the general adult and psychiatric intensive care units having done so on eight occasions in the preceding three months. On one of his escorted leaves, he had run off from his two escorts, entered a local shop, grabbed a bottle of vodka and as he raced out of the shop, snatched a lit cigarette out of the mouth of a passer-by before returning to the unit some hours later somewhat the worse for wear. We accepted him for admission because it seemed reasonable this degree of chaos was difficult to manage elsewhere. A protracted period of admission in a low secure unit might afford him the opportunity for medication compliance and keep him away from the dreaded drink. I didn't want to give him any leave for two weeks. This was extended to two months as he continued to be agitated, forever looking for a way out, checking the fence line and the movements of the staff. We had already arranged for the first tier tribunal panel to convene on the unit rather than at its usual place, as we were concerned Tom might abscond, particularly if the news was not to his liking. To their credit the panel agreed.

Tom however, began to settle. He seemed less agitated and was less thought disordered. Michaela gently suggested we had to take a risk. With a deep breath, we gave him some escorted leave, initially five minutes within the grounds with two male staff to be increased to 15 minutes, 30 minutes and so on. With each leave, Tom was reminded about the opportunity being presented to him, namely to demonstrate to himself and to us his ability to manage this increased responsibility. To his credit, and our surprise and relief, he didn't abscond. His leave is now increased with only one escort, either male or female and includes regular work at the Eden Project. He has now been transferred to Fettle, rehabilitation unit.

In retrospect, I was willing to co-operate with Michaela's suggestion, because although nervous, I trusted her, her experience, judgement and philosophy. Sarah and Pete agreed to be his escorts, and did so, because they knew they would have protected each other, were aware of each other and trusted each other. As Sarah commented "I wouldn't have picked anyone else to go with."

We also asked our new psychologist to contribute to this chapter. He wrote:

A psychologist's perspective

Positive risk taking doesn't always work out however, risk is a subject I find both fascinating and infuriating. Within the forensic world it seems to dominate, quite rightly, but I have been struck by the observation that the way clinical staff manage risk seems to have, on occasion, more to do with the personality and attitude of the clinician(s) than the history, behaviour and attitude(s) of the patient. While this idea is nothing new there may be a little mileage in outlining my own experiences in this area, both the good ones and the bad.

Before I decided to embark on the painfully long journey to become a clinical psychologist, I was lucky enough to work as a healthcare assistant (HCA) on various mental health and learning disability units. I remember quite clearly a visiting psychologist arriving one day to assess a particular patient, who I shall refer to as Barry, who had been quite challenging. As a result, he had earned a bit of a reputation amongst the staff team. While I don't remember the name of the psychologist, I do remember thinking there was little point in him talking to Barry as he was quite unwell at the time, and I thought he was likely to do this psychologist some damage. Anyway, after speaking to some of the other staff, the psychologist asked me (probably because I was known as psychology boy at the time) whether I would sit in on the assessment. I nervously agreed and we walked over to Barry's room. He was refusing to meet the psychologist in one of the interview rooms, as he believed those rooms had been bugged by MI5. Initially, as an HCA, I was surprised to be asked to sit in on the assessment but I was still more surprised at what happened next. After introducing himself to Barry who was already being quite oppositional, the psychologist asked if he could sit down. Barry said yes and the psychologist, rather than sitting on one of the two chairs within the room, instead sat down on the rather hard bedroom floor by the door.

I remember thinking this was really weird while at the same time also thinking if anything did happen he would struggle to get up from the floor in time before being walloped. However, my concerns were unfounded as Barry, rather than continuing to be aggressive, quickly relaxed and was actually able to express how he felt in a way I hadn't seen before. After the session had finished I asked the psychologist how he had done it. He described the importance of giving the patient space and listening to what they had to say rather than just asking questions that will confirm hypotheses we already hold true. He said he sat on the floor because it was the one of the best tools he knew to defuse mild aggression. He also told me that sitting on the floor in such a situation can be a very non-threatening physical gesture that is so far removed from what both staff and patients expect it creates an almost humorous/intriguing interest in both the psychologist and the assessment.

From a risk perspective I remember being struck by how the appropriate deployment of good clinical skills could not only defuse a potentially dangerous situation but also help a patient. Prior to this, both I and many of the other staff would avoid Barry when he was oppositional as we thought we would just aggravate the situation. I had never before thought Barry might actually be getting more annoyed because people didn't want to talk to him when he was upset.

While the above scenario has undoubtedly influenced my own views on risk, I like to think it also influences my clinical practice. During my last job I became aware that as a staff team we were often feeding patients lines such as "lets see how it goes" or "if you work with the team we will see what we can do." Such lines usually followed a patients request for leave following a recent 'risky' incident of some description. However, what those phrases do not tell patients is what they specifically need to do to get that increased leave and they can also lead to misunderstandings between patient and care team. For example, saying "if there are no more incidents in the next week, your leave will be increased" gives a patient something to aim for and a clear sense of what they need to do. While I am sure the clinical staff were aware of the importance of giving patients time limited goals, it is easy to lose sight of this in a busy unit environment where there are multiple and often competing demands on staff time.

The importance of using meaningful time limited goals in relation to positive risk taking is highlighted in the following case in which I was involved. The 20 year old gentleman in question (who shall be referred to as James), had an extensive forensic history for a man of his age and could be quite troublesome on the unit. He had a habit of obtaining and trading contraband, would regularly jam the locks with chewing gum, and could become violent towards staff. After spending some time getting to know James we somehow moved on to discuss the film 'Cliffhanger'. After thinking for a few moments

I offered James a slightly unorthodox clinical challenge. I asked firstly whether he fancied going indoor climbing and when he responded with a resounding 'yes', I said I would take him if he could remain incident free for three months.

While part of me secretly hoped I wouldn't have to come through with my promise, James managed to stay risk free for three months and enjoyed telling all and sundry he was going to make his psychologist climb the walls! When the day of reckoning came, James rose to the challenge (literally) and proved to myself and the instructor that not only could he behave impeccably but also that he was a great climber. While I look back favourably as I reminisce, at the time I was 'bricking it' so to speak and constantly questioned whether I had made the right choice and should have placed myself and James in a vulnerable position. While it was a carefully planned trip, it would have been easy not to offer the opportunity to James, it would also have been easy for James to jeopardise it at any point. I considered the trip a success because James had achieved a pro-social goal and in turn received the agreed although somewhat novel pro-social reward. However would the care plan have been seen as a success if the climbing trip itself had gone wrong in some way?

Shared responsibility and positive risk taking are terms I hear a lot about and aspire to work towards in a reasoned and managed way. However I have seen and been involved in situations when the above seemed to fall apart when things went pear shaped. While I understand the importance of investigating untoward incidents I feel it is important to allow for, and understand things can go wrong even if positive risks are taken in the right way for the right reasons. In particular, I feel it is important to protect those that make and take these appropriate positive risks for if it wasn't for these people positive change and recovery would be much slower if it happened at all. I suppose the point I am trying to make is when things do unfortunately go wrong, many staff feel the fickle finger of blame is trying to seek a fall guy. Even if there is no individual at fault the process staff go through often ensures no further positive risks are taken again.

I remember recently discussing this point with several members of the unit team while we were discussing what might be included in this book. I recalled how I was unfortunately involved in an incident which occurred on a community trip while I was working as an healthcare assistant. I described how myself and the others involved in the incident were subsequently reluctant to take further such risks in the future and how we blamed ourselves even though we couldn't fathom why it had happened. We saw the incident as some kind of negative reflection on us even though we were told there was nothing else we could have done.

Other staff in the meeting expressed they had had similar experiences and we discussed the importance of working with other staff you felt confident with. I suppose in a convoluted way, I am trying to promote an ideal that incidents can happen and making a mistake doesn't always have to be a bad thing. If James had gone AWOL on that climbing trip I have the unfortunate feeling the fact he had remained risk free for the previous three months would have been quickly forgotten."

To finish, we've included the following guiding statement and quotation:

"The Office of Mental Health acknowledges that making decisions about risk (together with service users and carers) are a part of everyday practice. The Office of Mental Health also recognises that clinicians are often faced with difficult dilemmas for which there is often no single or simple solution. The Office of Mental Health accepts the need for staff (and service users and carers) to arrive at these often high risk decisions and that not every decision taken has a successful or expected outcome. It supports the right and need for those decisions to be made. One means by which this can be achieved is by adherence to the tenets of good professional practice. The other is through the responsible use of a framework for safer practice and services for staff and users through the provision of sensible policy and protocol".

8 Whatever it takes

I had not worked in a rehabilitation service previously. From the outside it all seemed a bit slow and hopeless. It wasn't until I began to work on Bowman I could begin to have a sense of how hope can remain alive despite a long standing disadvantage that spans a person's life, and in turn, that of their families. You read about the importance of hope, but when I look at the recovery wheel, it's quite hard to know how you might develop a module around hopefulness, take it off the shelf as it were and incorporate it into a unit. I think that's why we wanted to include this chapter and name it because it might be that this is part of what makes Bowman work.

Again, it comes back to Michaela, the title being a phrase she used as we had begun to become despondent about increasingly trying to engage the men in activities. We went to the Community Meeting and the men suggested different activities like canoeing and kayaking, rock climbing and going to the cinema - all resource intensive activities off the unit and associated with a number of risks which needed to be considered. Michaela's view was simple "whatever it takes", and she meant it. "Find out about outdoor pursuits and if we need to get extra bank staff then we will". We did. Only one man went but as Michaela pointed out, it was important for that one man. It made a difference to him as an individual person. "Whatever it takes." I became enthusiastic about taking more men on a trip. Michaela commented she didn't want to return to "the bus load of patients going out on trips", an old institutional model. She wanted to replace this with individualised care. So if it meant we had to do more trips with one or two men at a time, then that's what we need to do. "Whatever it takes."

It also translated into the commitment of the staff. We were here during 'the big freeze' of 2010, or whatever it ends up being called! Much of the UK including Cornwall, was covered in snow. For our family, it was wonderful and novel. It was not how the staff approached the snow however. Michaela and Carol walked for two hours through snow in order to get to the unit. They realised the unit was likely to be short staffed and this placed everyone at risk. Some staff stayed overnight. Jess now knowing first hand how noisy and difficult it is to sleep there! Jason, in his 20s offered to take Joyce, in her 50s home as she lived out in the countryside caring for her husband. When he couldn't return, Joyce put him up for the night. Roster changes, visits, telephone calls of support, offers of part time work we all designed around staff helping each other out when personal circumstances became difficult. "Whatever it takes".

Another illustration of this is taking the time to celebrate arrivals, departures, birthdays and Christmas (each of the men receiving genuinely thoughtful gifts) and making sure all the staff on the day have the opportunity to sign cards. Little things that take time. Further examples include taking the men out to get the particular ingredients they want for their recipes, and making sure on takeaway nights there were a range of takeaways from which they could choose. This is all time consuming with separate trips, different menus and different amounts of money and change. There is also time taken for each of the men to choose their particular duvets, pictures and personal items for their room. 'Whatever it takes'.

Perhaps this "whatever it takes" philosophy contributed to the start of the outreach programme. Michaela had often observed in her previous job at a supported domestic house that although the team had been able to get people relatively settled they seemed to fall over as they were discharged. Although we're not quite sure what this is about, the idea of being able to follow our men as they took their initial steps into the community seemed worthwhile. The commissioners were generous and supported the costs of keeping the bed open for a month. Initially, we visited daily for two weeks, thrice weekly for the third week and twice in the fourth week.

One of our men was a bit disorganised, and although recognised staying off drugs and staying on medication was important, he forgot his morning tablets. When he began to relapse, we were able to recognise and manage his relapse while he stayed in the community by dispensing his daily medication from the unit. Fortunately he had settled into supported accommodation nearby, and it was interesting how he was almost in an institutionalised pattern of coming over each afternoon to pick up his medication. It also enabled Zach to keep in touch with the group of people he had spent the last two years with, and as such, a secure base. Even as his peers began to move on, it was important for Zach to keep coming over, have a cup of tea, a bit of a chat and to feel welcome. We also wondered whether or not he may have modelled to the other men it was possible to leave. Zach now manages his medication with his team and has been in supported accommodation for two years.

Whatever it takes.

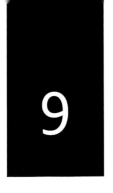

9 Medication

Laurence had been sent out of county for nearly 17 years with unremitting schizophrenia. In the few volumes of notes we had and from his discharge summary we noted he had been on Clozapine 950mg plus Risperidone 16mg, Olanzapine 20mg plus Droperidol 40mg, Risperidone 14mg plus Carbamazepine 400mg, Haloperidol 30mg, Chlorpromazine 1600mg, Zuclopenthixol Depot 400mg weekly plus Droperidol 80mg daily, Depakote 1300mg daily. Another man had been hospitalised for over 40 years of his life. After reviewing his 26 volume history, we noted there was no sustained relief but there was hypothyroidism and Grade III renal failure. Although discouraging, one of our friends sent us a list of treatments used many years ago. They included prescriptions for heroin, alcohol and cocaine for various ailments including cough, toothache and getting five day old infants to sleep! We don't know it all or get it right all of the time!

Medication is important. When I arrived on the unit for the first time, three things struck me in relation to medication. When I automatically assumed a required medication would have been an appropriate intervention, the staff gently introduced me to the unit culture which was one of talking, trying to understand what had happened that resulted in the distress and allowing time to recover and recompose.

The second observation was the somewhat daunting observation that most of the men were still unwell despite having taken the amount of medication they had been prescribed.

The third observation was for a small unit, two had experienced life threatening complications from clozapine which was identified early and corrected. Of course we had all read and known about these potential complications but I was aware of only one other person previously in my 20 year career to date. To find two people on the same unit who had definite and significant complications was striking. Given these three observations, I didn't quite know what to do. It was this that made me think perhaps the only thing I can do is to sit down and talk with the men.

I know it is a peculiar place to discuss talking under medication, but the effectiveness of talking did strike me as being remarkable. We had always been taught about the gene x environment interaction, 47% heritability with schizophrenia and John Wing's Three Hospital Study showing the benefits of a stimulating environment over a bland, 'one size fits all', institutional environment. To actually have the experience in front of you was remarkable.

Dean began to become interested in one of the young female staff and hostile towards the other men when she interacted with them rather than him. As he himself was young and of a similar age, it was a little unclear whether it was an understandable attraction on his part, or whether he may have been beginning to develop an erotomanic belief. We wanted to attend to this quickly. The team, including the female nurse, decided to sit down and to outline our concerns with Dean. He denied any feelings but the problem ended. Just like that. At first I didn't want to believe a 'psychosocial intervention' could be that effective, or more to the point, more effective than all of the medication tried to date. Yes, there are all sorts of other explanations. I began to look more carefully.

Another example is Laurence who had been on the medication listed above. I recognised the real possibility of Laurence being able to challenge his experiences. While sitting talking to me he described within an hour of arriving at the unit, that he was told by voices he would be executed if he entered his room. He entered his room. He then went on to describe the various animals inhabiting his body and as he spoke, he also told me a nurse was telling him they were entering his room and cutting off his face. He wiped his hand across his face and continued talking. He told me after 17 years of these and other experiences, he had taught himself to challenge and test those experiences and to stay with what he referred to as 'the basic facts.' "I'm sitting on a chair, I'm talking to the doctor. There's the door." I was in awe of his courage and again struck by the potential power of an intervention which had worked where medication had not.

Notwithstanding these intriguing observations, there is something in having the opportunity of being able to have a person on the unit for a protracted period of time, who has no access to illicit substances but can get regular medication. In contrast to the long list of medication this patient had been given, Tom responded to a simple regular depot. Dan, who had been initially conceptualised as having a personality disorder and a drug-induced psychosis, responded to Risperidone 5mg. Owen, for whom we were never quite sure about his diagnosis of schizophrenia, was well on Olanzapine 15mg. Simple, common, single antipsychotic medications, albeit in a contained and structured environment, could still be extraordinarily effective.

The more likely scenario, however was of men who had had many many attempts with medication which at best had partially treated their continuous, daily, persistent experiences. Sometimes we had some luck. I remember reading Mark's long medication history, and we are grateful to Linda, our pharmacist, who does an extraordinary job summarising and collating volume after volume of patient's notes in order to document their medication histories. It appeared, if he had responded to anything, it was Olanzapine 20mg and on a separate occasion Depixol 40mg. The problem however was significant weight gain - Mark weighed 131.4kg with a body mass index (BMI) of 43. On the basis of abnormal experiences, he remained assaultive, both verbally and physically and prior to transfer had been moving between the open acute admission unit and the psychiatric intensive care unit (PICU). Despite being thought disordered, Mark and I were able to discuss and consider the possibility of reintroducing each of these agents sequentially to see whether or not it might make a difference. Mark agreed and despite obvious psychosis, was able to continue this conversation over the next six to 12 months. We started with Olanzapine 10mg and watched for six months and measured any changes using the Brief Psychiatric Rating Scale. He began to recover and began to manage his weight differently. His improvement plateaued and as we had discussed, we added low dose Depixol, 10mg. Again further improvement followed. He now weighs 118kg, has not assaulted anyone and has been able to walk away from incidents that previously he may have reacted to differently. He is now on our open rehabilitation unit and has been for a year. It has been interesting sitting and talking to men who are clearly psychotic and yet able to have at times a considered discussion about medication.

What else to say about medication? Optimistically, I go to meetings and keep up-to-date hoping to find the treatment that will finally work. I am reassured if it were that clear and obvious, it would be out there. I am reminded of perhaps a little known fact that when electro-convulsive therapy (ECT) was first introduced in Europe, its use had spread to just over 40% of United States hospitals within three years. This occurred before television or the first global transfer of information on the internet. Its rapid and widespread use occurred because it was a successful treatment. While on the matter of biological treatments, it is probably worth putting in a note about ECT and schizophrenia. For acute exacerbations, ECT can be extraordinarily effective, albeit seldom used and having fallen into disfavour yet again. It is not so effective for chronic schizophrenia and therefore our population. We have tried the other little things like lamotrigine augmentation and fish oil as an Omega 3 supplement. The difficulty is a small sample size and as we have discussed elsewhere in this book, we are keen to link up with other low secure units in order to get a wider experience of our unique and pooled populations. I am not sure about lamotrigine. It seemed with one of our men, each 25mg increment seemed to be associated with a transient irritability. After four months, we decided to discontinue it as Dean was again becoming unwell. The difficulty was knowing whether this was due to medication, or whether it was because we were approaching Christmas, a difficult time for him. I think that's one of the other observations to make on a low secure unit. There is such an obvious combination of concurrent biological and psychosocial circumstances which are difficult to disentangle. Although large, pooled studies mitigate against this to some extent, they run the risk of glossing over individual phenomena. It might also be that some drugs require time, Clozapine and Olanzapine for example usefully require a six to 12 month trial before deciding whether or not they are effective. Maybe four months was too short.

The other thing we have been trying is buspirone. Having had a brief discussion with David, a professor of psychopharmacology who had come to give us a talk on a separate topic, I became interested in thinking about the psychopharmacological management of addiction and impulsivity. He suggested trying buspirone. There appeared to be an almost insatiable and voracious appetite for substances with some of our men. They will go to extraordinary lengths to obtain alcohol, illicit substances or indeed prescribed medications. Catch described one of her patients barging into the medication room, grabbing Lorazepam and fleeing. She leapt onto his back and tried to stop him from taking what she saw as her tablets! Help came quickly and the matter was managed.

We've already discussed Tom who while on escorted leave suddenly ran into the local shop, leant across the counter and grabbed a bottle of vodka. I am reminded of an animal experiment from my psychology days. I am somewhat cautious about introducing an animal model into a book about people, but I have done so on this occasion to illustrate the point. Upon stimulation a mouse kept pressing a lever which had no particular function other than it was paired previously to food release. The mouse continued to press the lever without pausing, without taking time for food or water and without sleep. This illustrated to me the overriding drive for what is thought to be a pleasurable experience and what they refer to as 'an independent pleasure centre'. This overrode any other aspects of their lives. It made me think about the possibility, that our men may not have control. If their pre-existing psychosis is exacerbated by illicit substances, they really are significantly disabled.

Previously, perhaps to manage my own anxiety by obsessionality, I have tried to stay with one medication, increase it to a maximumally tolerated dose, before reducing, stopping and sequentially trialling the next agent. Too often I have found combinations of medication unhelpful in trying to delineate which had and had not been effective, and therefore, what to continue and what to simplify. When I was a locum in Tasmania, the director, Mani, very usefully introduced me to Stahl's Essential Psychopharmacology. I began to think about multiple receptors being involved in schizophrenia. Therefore targeting those specific receptors with a combination of antipsychotics rather than relying on one alone might be useful. For some reason, not the least of which was Mani's gentle and encouraging manner, I decided to try this. The theory also gave me a potential medico-legal defence should it all go pear shaped! It also provided hope and enthusiasm and therefore a renewed interest in matters psychopharmalogical. When I arrived at Bowman Unit where some of the men were typically on a number of different antipsychotics, I began to ask them about their experiences. Again, and to my surprise, both they and the staff recognised the addition of amisulpride to clozapine was useful. Patients of course talk, and Jon came up and asked for the same. He too reported a benefit, although I was less impressed by it myself and declined his requests for higher and higher doses.

The other thing I came across, again from talking to the men, was the use of clonidine for extrapyrimidal side effects. As you might imagine various anticholinergic agents including benztropine, procyclidine and orphenadrine had been tried as had beta-blockers. Jon had responded to a depot, Pipotiazine palmitate 50mg fortnightly, and although his extra-pyramidal side effects were less, they were still quite marked. As there was an anxiety component I added in an SSRI. I later read one line in an article on extra pyramidal side effects that suggested SSRIs could exacerbate this side effect. Indeed it had as Jon was barely able to hold a cup of tea. He was very agreeable as I apologised to him for 'inadvertently poisoning him' and although it had helped his anxiety, it may have worsened his tremor. He took it in good faith and we discontinued the SSRI. In the context of this ongoing working relationship, Jon raised the suggestion of clonidine which he had been on previously. I was concerned but read and thought a therapeutic trial was not unreasonable. It worked! You know what I'm going to say of course, yes, always listen to your patients! Funny how you never stop learning and sometimes re-learning those things you are already supposed to have learnt! Maybe that too has been the benefit of working on a unit where the men have seemingly 'all had treatment resistant schizophrenia'. There is still space to sit and talk with people, with sometimes the most amazing results.

So what are my thoughts on medication? Its effectiveness can be elegant in its simplicity. Smaller doses of drugs that have previously been effective, occasionally in combination with a patient approach can make a difference that enables at least some of the men to move to a less secure setting. Continuing to explore possibilities by observing and incorporating different literatures maintains a hopefulness that can be shared with men who have a persistent psychosis. It's a tricky old field with that gene x environment interaction. It is difficult to partial out one effect from another, but also fascinating that psychosocial interventions can be so extraordinarily effective, either singly or in combination with medication. Again we would be interested in your observations.

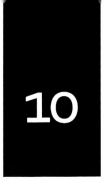

10   "We know best"

We can feel some people cringe as they read that heading! We know it's a bit provocative but interestingly, there is an element of truth in it as well. We think the trick is in finding the balance between two competing ethical principles, paternalism and autonomy. We looked up paternalism on the internet recently and want to quote this.

> "Paternalism has become a politically unpopular word because of its association with physicians telling patients what is good for them, without regard to the patient's own need and interest. This limited sense of paternalism is improper and has been obviated by informed consent requirements. In the larger sense, however, the relationship between medical care practitioners and patients is a paternalistic, beneficent relationship: medical care practitioners are expected to do what is medically best for the patient. ...it never includes improper medical care given only because the patient requests it. Despite the importance of patient involvement and informed consent, medical care practitioners are expected to do what is best for their patient. In certain public health situations,

they are also expected to consider what is best for society, even if that may not be in the best interests of the patient."

If we were able to attribute this to somebody we think it was the Low Secure Unit Medical and Public Health Law site written by Professor Edward Richards. This explanation introduces balance and common sense to the area. It is difficult to be the responsible team which argues for the continued detention of a person, and where seemingly simple requests such as a walk in the hospital grounds requires consideration, and at times, may seem like a denial of basic rights. Yet, men who have been restricted, have also had the opportunity of recovery because those same restrictions have been a useful adjunct to their treatment.

We think the challenge is being able to begin to share the responsibilities, or to use some of the language in the literature, develop a partnership rather than a paternalistic relationship alone. There's now a new Salzburg Statement on shared decision making. In some ways it is linked to our section on 'positive risk taking' for this is what partnerships and power sharing, (or whatever the phrase might be), is about. While "we may know best", we also need to be able to offer the person an opportunity to take on new responsibilities and show to themselves and to us, life can change. The difficulty is when a lot is seemingly at stake. We think we try and do this by again being clear with the men.

Tom for example, each and every time he went out on his escorted, then gradually his unescorted leave, was reminded this was an opportunity to show responsibility both for himself and to us. With that demonstration he could progress to greater leave, greater opportunities and a real chance of being able to leave the unit. He was subsequently able to thank us for that responsibility.

Another illustration of this we wanted to raise was Mr A who we discharged, but had relapsed and returned. Mr A would often come up to us and ask whether he could go on leave. It felt as if he was asking his parents for something. We responded by falling into the pattern of either agreeing or refusing his leave. We began to invite Mr A to consider whether or not he might be well enough to have his leave and discuss this with us, instead of asking permission. He did. He recognised he didn't feel well enough to go into town, and stopped asking. Two or three days later his experiences began to settle and he went on leave.

We made a lot of this to him, namely his own ability to monitor and regulate his mental state for his leave. Similarly we were able to engage him in trialling depot medication. Mr A reminded us he had discontinued his oral medications on two previous occasions and this led to his return to hospital. He could see taking depot medication would not only be helpful to his community treatment team who would know his medication was being reliably delivered, but that he himself could be reassured. He accepted the co-administration of his oral and depot medication. Each was a low dose, but seemed to help, with minimal side effects. There was a significant change - Mr A had learnt a different way to manage his relapses. At the age of 21 maybe this will hold him and the team in good stead as we continue to meet him over the next 40 years.

We know we are supposed to do work on the index offence. We understand that if together we are able to explore the circumstances of the offence, we may be able to better support the person and thereby prevent a recurrence. However, after 20 odd years we could also understand Paul's view. It was such a long time ago. He'd been over it lots of times in the past and didn't want to discuss it any further. We could appreciate this was a difficult area for him and we weren't convinced 'badgering the witness' would necessarily be helpful. What was interesting was by not attending to his index offence, putting it to one side and gently continuing by enabling his supportive transfer to Fettle House (rehabilitation unit), led to an important request.

Paul wanted to visit the grave of his grandmother, with whom his index offence had arisen, in order to pay his respects. He recognised this would be difficult to do with his mother. As he had formed a close relationship, over many years, with his forensic community psychiatric nurse (FCPN), Debbie, he chose to do this with her, privately and without fuss. Maybe this was Paul's way of beginning to genuinely look at his index offence. Paul knew best!

So, who knows best? Each of us contribute and offer something to the relationship. It's a matter of respecting and acknowledging sometimes the 'other' does know best.

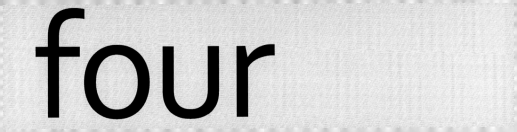

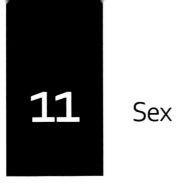

11 Sex

Male desires, female staff

Mel was a young, healthcare assistant who had come from caring for the elderly who were often confused and required a lot of nursing. It involved quite a different approach to the men on Bowman who she described as "being real men with real feelings and real hormones."

Like me, Mel felt sorry for one of the young men, but also found him intimidating and hadn't wanted to 'trip that switch with him'. Mel wanted to try and involve the men, using her bubbly personality to get them up, get them involved and, included in society. She loved the fact she could go out with them on escorted leave and try and get them reconnected with their community.

However this enthusiasm changed. The chap seemed to target Mel: "Can I have a chat with you? I like spending time with you. I like it best when you go on leave with me" and began to smile at her and became uncomfortable when she was talking with the other men. Mel knew he was 'hitting on her'. She started to ask him not to say those things. That it wasn't right, and you shouldn't do that, but she knew it was too late. She became aware she didn't want to be on her own with him. She only wanted to interact with him when she was in a communal setting with others around, and was frightened she would be put into a position where things might go wrong. Eventually she went to Catch and said "I can't do this."

As mentioned earlier in the book, we sat down as a team with both Mel and the young man and addressed this issue directly. Sadly, and because we were frightened of the possibility this was unable to be managed by this intervention alone, we thought it was safer for Mel to be shifted to another unit. Regrettably, Mel felt she had been punished. Fortunately it transpired the unit where she had been sent was our psychiatric intensive care unit (PICU) where boundaries are clear, defined and implemented as part of the culture of managing a unit which at times can become quite disturbed. Mel now recognises the changes she has made as a result, she enjoys working there and has recently been accepted for nursing training. She has met the young man in the street two or three times and it is interesting he has been content to just say hello and to keep walking. Maybe our intervention had been effective.

When we asked Mel what she would do differently, she said she wished she had gone to one of the nurses earlier and had dealt with it more quickly. She is also aware she has changed in terms of being clear, direct and honest with a person - laying the ground rules and meaning it.

As a team we learnt as the following account from Lisa illustrates.

Lisa, a young, student nurse had recently joined the unit for a six month attachment. The experience she had and she describes below captures part of managing male desires with a mixed gender staff group.

Lisa

A dream I always remember having was that I used to want to be a solicitor; I recently remember reading an old school report where I had a work placement for ten days in a solicitor's office. I must've been 15 years old (I can already hear some huffing that that wasn't even ten years ago I know) but for me that was a long time ago. I can't really think of what made me change my mind. I then found another report where I decided I wanted to be some sort of psychologist, with those being my exact words. But never has nursing entered the equation - let alone mental health nursing. If I'm completely honest, I didn't realise I wanted to even be a mental health nurse until 2008, and by then I was a year into my course. Each of us has challenges. For me, in my final year I was naive to think mine were over, (well at least within the course) and the only challenges I would face for my final six months would be getting my coursework done and dusted and gaining the confidence to present a powerpoint presentation and taking part in a viva or interview. To me, that was the biggest obstacle I was going to face. I had for some reason ignorantly developed the idea that a 6 month placement in Bowman, a low secure unit would not set me any further challenges, except the usual you face in each placement, meeting new staff, fitting in with a new team, new patients and a new area of mental health, which are to me not challenges, but stepping stones to creating who I become when I qualify. Although this area of mental health was completely new to me, I genuinely couldn't think of anything that would seriously challenge me enough to make me question who I am (as a nurse) and whether I was right for mental health nursing. But all the same I couldn't wait - experience in forensic mental health, a low secure unit. I was one of the lucky ones in my class to get such an exciting placement for my final months of training.

On starting on the unit I was not surprised, but comforted by the fact every one was so friendly and welcoming. It's natural to feel nervous in any new place, but on starting placements there is not always an opportunity to meet the team before you start. So you're almost walking in blind. Within weeks I was settled and felt like a valued member of the team. The idea of entering an all male unit didn't faze me at all. Although it was my first experience of a single sexed unit, over the years of training I had become more comfortable working with males then I had expected, and as yet, had never felt intimidated or uncomfortable in their presence.

After a few weeks a new guy was admitted to the unit. On greeting this patient, I was one of the first members of staff to meet him, I was pleasant and he was friendly and appropriate.

After a few days this patient seemed to be settling well. He was polite in interactions, and telling us information about himself. I then started to notice this patient was making comments towards me that made me feel uncomfortable. At first I dismissed the first few comments of "you have lovely hair" and "you look nice today" as being his way of settling in with new staff and surroundings, I didn't really pay any attention to it as other members of staff, mainly female, had reported similar comments.

One day when I was in the pool room with another patient. He was in there watching and started saying these things again, but some of the questions/comments started to become more personal. While playing pool I suddenly became very aware he was behind me and he then asked me if I had a tattoo on my stomach. My first thoughts when he asked this was 'crap, my top has shifted'. However on checking it hadn't. I then thought 'I haven't got any tattoos, so even if my top had moved, it wouldn't have shown a tattoo of any kind. I said to him "No,

I didn't have a tattoo but your comment is inappropriate". He then said staff at a previous unit had had tattoos, implying he had either intentionally been shown these, or unintentionally seen these. He continued to ask me questions, private personal questions about myself that made me feel uncomfortable. Although at this point I was not completely freaking out, I did make an effort to let other staff know what had been said but without completely stating it had made me feel uneasy. During a meeting between this patient and our psychologist, my name was mentioned by him and in a way that was unrelated to the work they were doing. I decided to just become more vigilant with any future interactions. It wasn't until I worked a weekend shift where I started to become more concerned about this particular patient and his interaction with me. I suddenly started to become afraid of being on my own with him on the unit in case he approached me again. I felt he had already cornered me in a corridor to make the remark that I reminded him of his ex-wife. While at times patients do invade our personal space, this can usually be solved by just taking a step back and discussing it with them. For some reason this was not happening and I became more uncomfortable.

I started to dwell on it when I was at home. I was really confused. I didn't know what to do. I also had nobody to talk to at home about it as

I didn't know if I was over-reacting. I had no reassurances. By this time I knew myself this was a problem. It was starting to interfere with who I was and how I worked.

When I returned after the weekend, and before the unit round, I took the other student to one side. In one way I wanted her to say I was over-reacting, but on the other I hand I wanted someone to completely agree. After a lengthy conversation, she said she could tell by my tone and body language this really bothered me. The fact I had been thinking about it all weekend was another sign this was serious. Although I had already planned in my head to talk to Michaela, I now knew that I would. I don't like talking in front of large groups of people, and although I had had the above conversation I still felt afraid of letting other team members know how much this was bothering me. As stupid as this may sound, I suddenly really felt my age. I felt that after three years of hard work, long, busy and mentally draining placements, constantly trying to prove that although young I was old and strong enough to cope, I suddenly felt like I was simply a little girl. As I sat through unit round I was losing my confidence planning in my head what I was going to say and to whom. Could I say it in front of Dr Little? Would the other team members think this was a complete over reaction? Would Michaela and Iain be annoyed I had just brought it up in the unit round without letting them know first? What was worse, there was no knowing if there would be consequences for this and how it may effect the rest of my placement. I just didn't know.

At the end of the unit round I had made my decision and before everyone got up to leave I simply said I would like to talk about this particular person. What a relief it was to just talk about the problem openly. I knew then there was no retracting it and I had to follow through. Suddenly everyone's eyes were on me. I felt sick waiting for the response. Although I had no doubts the team would be anything but supportive, if I am honest, there was a very small part of me wondered if they thought, young girl, on an all male unit, over-reacting a little bit. This was not the case at all. Each and every person in the room was 100% supportive. I couldn't have asked for a better response. What was even more supporting was that they asked me what I wanted to happen. I had no idea. I wasn't too sure what I wanted to do about it, what was best for me and what was best for that patient also. We talked about it as a team and agreed the female staff on the unit would sit and talk with this patient and let him know his behaviour was inappropriate and needed to stop, but without me speaking or the group indicating it was me who had raised the concern.

Interestingly there were mixed views amongst

the staff. Some felt he didn't realise how inappropriate he had been, some had commented they had not felt uncomfortable despite similar comments and some had asked why they hadn't been complimented. Others including myself, felt he was aware of the inappropriateness of his behaviour. The patient said he was just making 'banter', but stopped anyway.

I would be lying if I said this hadn't affected me. I was very confused thinking I may have encouraged this, even without realising which really set me back a bit. I also subconsciously think sometimes my interactions with patients are guarded but with this particular patient, I don't feel my interactions have changed or are any different had this not happened. Time will tell.

Sexual dysfunction

Mr A is a young 21 year old man who came to our unit. Amongst other things, he was concerned about what he called his "sexual dysfunction". We thought about this in terms of his medication; Mr A often cited sexual dysfunction as a legitimate reason for its discontinuation. Mr A explored the internet himself and found a drug that was less likely to do this. We tried it but it resulted in a worsening in his clinical condition. We also noted, that when he was re-admitted but wasn't on medication, he was still complaining of 'sexual dysfunction'. Despite his age we explored the obvious diseases, including diabetes and hypertension. We asked whether or not he was able to get a morning erection, which would confirm his biological function was intact. We also thought about this as being part of his relapse signature. Mr A was concerned about a number of physical symptoms including his sexual functioning which had heralded many previous relapses and admissions. However going through his story again, there were one or two notes in the many volumes which alluded to the possibility his mother may have molested him as a young child. We suggested to Mr A psychological aspects to his sexual dysfunction. He initially dismissed these but then he considered the idea and 'wanted counselling'. For some reason, I can't recall, I felt out of my depth again. How do you do instigate orientated psychotherapy with a person who has schizophrenia? Would it make things worse? I was unsure about it.

Mr A however asked to go to the GU clinic where he had been previously. He wanted to get some information, and although we had given this to him, he was unable to be reassured. While he may have had three orgasms a day when he was younger, this changes with age. The GU clinic, despite offering this service to people without schizophrenia, felt it was an inappropriate referral. Perhaps they were also scared. The issue of his sexuality was raised but Mr A dismissed this. He felt, while he may have had fleeting homosexual thoughts, he was heterosexual. He did acknowledge he had difficulty knowing how to relate to women but he was interested in females. Finally, we began to consider why there was such a persistent preoccupation with his sexual capacity, despite being able to achieve satisfactory orgasm on most days. We then began to think about Mr A's sexual functioning as a metaphor for his potency. So much of his life had been lost, so much ability to control his own destiny had been lost, and once again he found himself powerless in a locked secure unit with an uncertain future. An ability to get an erection, to be a man, afforded Mr A the opportunity of regaining power, control and mastery over at least this part of his life. Once understood and labelled, the issue started to evaporate.

Gender dysphoria

Simon was a young man on our unit who was doing well. In addition to his index offence and schizophrenia, Simon wanted to have a sex change. schizophrenia, a forensic history and now a sex change was a bit daunting for me having just started in the unit and I put it to one side. However things don't go away. I've included a copy of my letter to an NHS Gender Dysphoria Clinic to let you know what happened subsequently.

Simon

Dear Sir

Re: Simon

I first met the above named in my capacity as a locum general adult psychiatrist on a low secure unit in Cornwall. At the time of my arrival, the majority of the work was in relation to his initial illness, schizophrenia complicated by illicit substance use, and his index offence had largely been resolved. Accordingly I facilitated his transfer to Fettle House, an open rehabilitation unit on the Bodmin Hospital site. While I remained aware of his ambivalence regarding his gender, I had not seen this as a primary issue.

Unfortunately, Simon's treating psychiatrist at Fettle House became unwell and was absent for a period of time and I was asked to assist. In this revised role, one of the matters that was important for Simon was his gender and whether he should or should not proceed to irreversible surgical intervention. I discussed with him my limited knowledge of this area but was happy to explore aspects of it and to refer him to a speciality clinic such as yours for review and consideration. Rather than doing this without thought or enquiry, I spent some weeks exploring some limited aspects of his wish to consider transgender surgery.

What struck me was Simon's capacity to consider parts of the problem. I had asked him to write a developmental timeline from when he first thought about possibilities and discovered these both predated his definable mental illness and continued after its relative resolution and in the absence of illicit drugs. Simon reported to me that he had previously been seen by a gender dysphoria clinic in London, had taken feminising hormones and had intermittently been in the role of a female, including dressing as a woman while on Fettle and in the local community.

What was also evident, and as discussed with Simon, was a long standing ambivalence stretching over several years, which suggested that his request for gender reassignment was not straightforward or clear to himself.

When I asked Simon to think about his sexuality, who and what he might be sexually excited by and with whom he might wish to have a sexual relationship, his near 12 page developmental timeline was reduced to a single paragraph. Within this paragraph Simon himself was able to recognise that his sexuality was unclear and he regarded himself as 'asexual'. He ventured the statement that he wanted to be treated in the way that men treat women, finding them attractive, companionable and of seeking and receiving nurture. Simon was reluctant to explore this further, commenting that he was concerned that any further exploration might jeopardise his chances for irreversible surgery. In an attempt to clarify his resolve, I invited Simon himself to write to his former clinic seeking his old notes and asking for an NHS based clinic that was closer to the South West. He has been able to do this, but perhaps without the same vigour. On a subsequent visit, while having completed his homework, the issue relating to his gender and sexuality once again seemed to fade as it has over the years and we began to focus on other aspects of his rehabilitation and return to the community, which included budgeting and accommodation options.

My colleague returned and I returned Simon to her care. However I felt an obligation to honour my original position to explore with him the possibility of gender reassignment, to acknowledge his dysphoria and ambivalence and to refer him to an NHS based service for further consideration and review.

Accordingly I would be grateful if you would see Simon and would be interested in your approach and recommendations.

I have given Simon a copy of this letter.

Yours faithfully

Dr John Little
Locum Consultant Psychiatrist

cc Simon

Although Simon has successfully moved onto Fettle, rehabiliation unit and then out to a supported house in the community, he still has his copy of the letter and will send it when he feels ready.

Pornography

Sex is part of human nature and therefore part of the dynamic which occurs in any human organisation. Addressing any number of issues that may arise requires an open, honest acknowledgement as to its existence, subsequent consideration and discussion before managing it directly. Again the men had interesting, thoughtful and surprisingly realistic views about this area. We have included them in our appendices of community meetings.

We've thought about sex and our men. Aside from the immediate and obvious logistical difficulties, there is

also something else. Our men have lost so much of what other people may take for granted. The opportunity of enjoying a sexual relationship is another loss our men, who are likely to remain in hospital for many years, will also experience. It is a sad part of life.

12 Drugs and alcohol

Alcohol has been a 'chestnut' on the unit and I'm still not sure we've got it right. Obviously some of the men had difficulties and for a few it was relatively clear they should never drink again. Others had difficulties but seemed to make a career out of them. Others still were not particularly interested.

We wanted to give the men an opportunity to behave responsibly with their escorted and eventually unescorted leave. I used to become quite angry when, having taken a risk, someone would come back having had one or two cans. Why would you jeopardise all you have gained for the sake of a few drinks? I questioned why I would put my name onto a leave form and suffer the consequences if it all went wrong. Why not just forbid all alcohol and suspend all leave? Paul was quite helpful. He said one of the things he likes about working on Bowman Unit is that we continue to give men a chance. It may have been Catch who added it takes some 78 attempts before the penny drops. I think it was the acceptance of relapse and the not giving up on the men which impressed me.

As with other slightly contentious issues, we wanted to

discuss it at the community meeting so the men could be involved in planning how we might manage alcohol breaches. It was interesting to get their perspective. They felt if you drunk on one occasion, you should lose all leave for a week; two occasions and lose it for a month; and three occasions lose the leave for three months. While it was both interesting and useful to have the support of the men in terms of trying to manage the use of alcohol, there was a certain uneasiness as well. This could easily spiral into an increasingly punitive stance on our part, where some men might end up without any leave at all. We decided to get some help.

Combined Bowman Unit Low Secure Unit and Community Forensic Team meeting in relation to developing an alcohol policy for Bowman Unit

15 October 2009

Attached:

1. Contribution from the Bowman Unit Community Meeting dated 10 September 2009 with input from Service Users.
2. Support Plan and Outcome Star Guide
3. Letter to Cornwall Drug and Alcohol Team (CDAT)

Background:

- Presently there are a number of patients on Bowman Unit whose primary psychiatric diagnosis has been significantly complicated by alcohol and drug use.
- There is agreement that alcohol and drugs are not

included on Bowman Unit. As patients move on however, there is then an opportunity for returning to substance use and abuse. It is thought that rather than an 'all or none' approach, consideration be given to providing patients with an opportunity to explore responsible drinking in a considered and graduated manner.

- It was also noted that there are a number of the present patients who entered the mental health system from the age of 15 onwards at a time when their personalities were still forming and that they may have had little opportunity to develop appropriate alcohol use, this being affected by both their youth and the erosion of their personality by the schizophrenic process itself.
- Recently one of the Bowman patients had been tested in the community in a nightclub setting during an escorted leave. Useful feedback was provided by the Community Forensic Team at the time, prompting this meeting for a review of the policy.

Positive Risk Taking

- There was unanimous agreement amongst those present for recognition that managing alcohol appropriately was important. It was acknowledged that although the safest option was to forbid all alcohol or any testing of alcohol use in the community, that ultimately this was unrealistic and potentially left the person at the point of discharge ill equipped for assuming the responsibilities associated with that discharge to a less secure setting.
- It was further thought that within the framework of a low secure environment, positive risk taking with due consideration and appropriate management and contingency plans were an important part of the rehabilitation cycle.

- Further, in other low secure units contacted there was an absence of an alcohol policy and that together we could formulate a set of guidelines that could be 'fine tuned' and developed over time. Fettle House, rehabilitation unit were interested in attending in order that there might be a consistent approach linking rehabilitation in this part of east Cornwall.

Appropriate Assessment

- Thought would need to be given to individualised care packages. For some patients, being identified for alcohol abstinence was the most appropriate course of action. Others however, may be able to learn from a measured and appropriate use of alcohol in a graduated fashion. The identification of which patient falls into which category is important.

- As a continuation of the general group based current alcohol programme on the unit. Education about alcohol as a destabilising factor while being a culturally valued activity amongst the broader community. There are also health and duty of care considerations in relation to binge drinking, plus long-term consequences both psychiatric and general physical health plus the alcohol withdrawal policy including the prevention of long-term brain damage to be considered.

- In terms of being able to offer an individualised package for identified patients, invitations will be extended to agencies either on an inreach or outreach capacity including Cornwall Alcohol and Drugs Agency (CADA) and Alcoholics Anonymous (AA).

- Thought was given to inviting Cornwall Drug and Alcohol Team (CDAT) to educate not only the patients but also our staff, on how to manage individualised care packages specifically focused on alcohol would be useful.

- Consideration be given to identifying and supporting a staff member on Bowman Unit to develop a specialist portfolio in relation to alcohol.

- Individualised care packages will include an understanding of common pathways to alcohol use. This could include cultural expectations, anxiety management, enjoying violence but managing this except when disinhibited by alcohol, binge drinking. It is accepted each facet may require a slightly different and targeted approach depending on the person's unique difficulties and needs.

- In addition to enhancing competency to manage difficulties, thought also needs to be given to enhancing the motivation to remain abstinent. Suggestions included providing feedback on liver transamanaise; particularly gamma GT and the 'Quick Drinkers Check Up' by Miller and Risnick (around 1985) may provide a quick and ready cognitive feedback to the person on the affects of alcohol.

- Medication options including the use of acamprosate, disulfiram or naltrexone.

- A note was also made that patients on Section 37/41 may have, as part of their restrictions, complete abstinence from alcohol. This also needs to be considered in terms of developing a suitable plan.

- Any individual care plan in which escorted and unescorted leave, is part of the rehabilitation and recovery programme, there is a specific focus on alcohol. Therefore rather than it being just an outing to the pub, because there are staff available and interest has been expressed, there is a specific focus. The patient goes to the pub with a trained staff member. Initially this may be for a meal without alcohol and to explore urges and feelings and how they are managed, the use of nonalcoholic drinks and if successful, gradually increased to shandys, low alcohol beer and possibly full strength depending on progress or lack thereof.

- Such a targeted plan would be one of the filaments of the rehabilitation and recovery star (attached) which could then travel with the person at discharge should that be Fettle House rehabilitation unit or into the community.

- Equally should the person be linked into an AA or CADA programme, and then the sponsor would become part of the potential social support network as the person moves into the community.

Sanctions?

- In the real world, there is a process over ten or so years where all of us have the experience of being able to use alcohol and to self correct. This happens either by direct feedback or from the observations of what has happened to others in our network of family and friends. This may include losing jobs, losing relationships and over a period of time, as we mature, we learn what is an appropriate use of alcohol for ourselves.

- Unfortunately, and particularly for those people who have entered the mental health system at a young age, this normal maturation process is unavailable. Further, alcohol may be a way of signalling to the treatment team their ambivalence and/or opposition to their protracted and involuntary admissions.

- Although the patients on Bowman Unit had spontaneously suggested an increase in sanctions, with each occasion of alcohol use, the concern was this may become increasingly restrictive and ultimately counter productive with patients spending protracted periods of time without leave.

- Increasing restrictions also may reflect counter transference hatred which would need to be managed individually, in supervision, in the reflective practice group or elsewhere.

- The suggestion was made that rather than restricting leave in an incremental fashion, consideration be given to converting unescorted leave back to escorted leave. During escorted leave, there is a specific focus on alcohol use. 'Drink urge diaries' would also be used in an attempt to document a chain analysis of thoughts and feelings that may lead to alcohol use. Pairing of a diary with a pub experience may also be an aversive experience.

- The rationale and message therefore is not one of sanctions in which the treatment team is taking responsibility. Rather it invites, encourages and supports the person to see alcohol as being a task they have to manage. For many alcohol has led to a series of difficulties in their life including protracted compulsory admission, leave restrictions as well as health consequences.

Other Matters

- Education of staff was again highlighted. An invitation was extended to CDAT to assist the Bowman staff in terms of appropriately assessing and identifying which patients fell into which category. For example complete abstinence or controlled drinking as well as providing a skill set so any staff member, who is taking a person on escorted leave is appropriately equipped. This allows the staff member to engage the person and encourage them to manage alcohol themselves. There is a clear focus on exploring urges and motivations for alcohol use so alternatives can be identified, explored and tested.

- Whilet staff are being trained in motivational interviewing, the long term cognitive effects of both schizophrenia at a young age as well as polysubstance abuse may make it difficult for the person, who impulsively absconds and drinks, seemingly with little capacity, to pause, reflect and consider consequences and change direction.

- Once the policy is in place and developing, consideration will be given to writing to the Ministry of Justice so they are aware of the Bowman Low Secure Unit approach to alcohol.

- As part of the treatment programme, lots of praise and reinforcement will be given even for seemingly small achievements such as walking past a pub without having any urge.

- In relation to one patient, the notion of 'pathological drinking' was noted. Although the veracity of this as a clinical syndrome was unclear as well as ethically and logistically difficult to test, despite the secure setting Bowman might offer.

- Having asked the patients themselves at the Community Meeting, where they came up with the accumulating sanctions, that this be acknowledged and as part of an ongoing process. Reviews and different approaches to be discussed in the community meeting to avoid the potential problem of democratic apathy, namely 'you asked, we told you what we thought and yet you changed and did your own thing anyway so why ask us?'.

End Note

I discussed the above possibility with one of our young men. He said he didn't want anything to do with it and would rather miss out on any leave than put up with this.

Always a dilemma!

Dr John Little
Locum Consultant Psychiatrist

As a result John, a Forensic Psychologist, did speak to us. He enabled us to reflect about alcohol in a broader context and to begin to see our unit as a 'mini society' with a culture within which alcohol is part and parcel of everyday life. David, a Consutant in Drugs and Alcohol also visited and we developed a link with his service:

Letter to David

Dear David

First of all, thank you very much for coming along to Bowman Unit yesterday having both braved the conditions and done a background search on the internet for matters relevant to our specific population. I am also personally grateful for you changing your appointment at the last minute.

I thought I would dictate this letter, in part to collect some of the ideas and also to document the process as it unfolds. I only wish I had taken a few more notes at the time, but here goes!

I think it is important to note there was considerable interest amongst the staff in attending today and despite the phones ringing, the doorbell being pressed and the other requirements on the unit, all the available staff on the day were able to attend for at least part of the time. Present were Michaela, Mark, Jason, Carol, Will, Karen and myself.

In no particular order:

1. What evidence was available suggested a 12 step unit based programme was likely to be unsuccessful.

2. Individualised care packages attending to the specific needs of people on a person by person basis seemed to be the most effective.

3. Your own experience with agents such as Antabuse involves fully informed consent without coercion. This was in a community based clinic with an acknowledgement that an inpatient forensic population may require different approaches. I was vaguely aware of an article comparing enforced treatment with offenders compared to 'treatment as usual' with the benefit of the former. I will try to explore this on the internet with respect to community treatment orders (CTOs) imposed conditions which may include the supervision and administration of Antabuse or other agents and whether or not that has been successful.

4. We are particularly pleased with the offer of a referral mechanism to Cornwall Drug and

Alcohol Team (CDAT) with a case based learning approach. We appreciate you have a 21 day response time. Accordingly we will take our referrals to Matt who has a fortnightly clinic on the Bodmin site. As you noted this is an important opportunity to build bridges between our two services and certainly we would be happy to come and talk to your team at any time should that be felt to be useful. Over time we would hope therefore that either with rotating staff attending Matt's clinic or with a follow-up meeting to discuss individuals, the broader Bowman team will have an opportunity to up skill and to continue in the development of our approach towards the management of significant drug and alcohol issues within our population.

5. An educational programme post detoxification may also be useful, not withstanding most of our men have been detoxified before transfer. It might be useful for one or more of us to attend on invitation to see whether or not it is relevant for our group.

6. Michaela in particular spoke highly of both Katie and Hazel in terms of their skill at pitching their teaching to the level of the audience. She found them to be enthusiastic speakers and again this would be a useful addition to the development of alcohol and drug management on our unit.

7. We are also pleased to learn that the possibility of after-care at discharge may continue with yourselves or onward referral to AdAction, previously known as Cornwall Alcohol and Drug Agency (CADA).

Opinion
While I tried to list the various elements I recalled, I think the more important part was your gentle nature and willingness to contribute to an ongoing developmental process on the unit. With shared input between our two teams, and with individualised case based discussions, it will be interesting to see how it unfolds. Once again I am most grateful for your interest in involvement and hopefully this will establish a good working relationship.

Dr John Little
Locum Consultant Psychiatrist

So where are we left with alcohol?

I became more interested in the issues surrounding drugs and alcohol. I started to do some reading and wondered whether or not I should visit some specialist units. Crisping up our approach to both drugs and alcohol would be an important part of our rehabilitation programme. It covers one of the filaments of the recovery star and one of the clinical risk items for the HCR-20 (risk assessment tool). I began to think about what specialist units might offer that is different to Bowman. My assumption is that their culture may focus on drugs and alcohol. Ours is more broadly focused on rehabilitation, recovery and return to the community. There is also an excellent educational article in the American Journal of Psychiatry (2010) which we've included in the references. It's not that it 'has the answer', rather it provides an approach for a General Adult Psychiatrist, such as myself, to become acquainted with new pharmacological understandings and suggestions to rekindle hopefulness and an approach other than despair.

Recently I thought a friend of the family had a significant alcohol problem. It transpired matters were more complicated than they had first appeared. Nevertheless, having been asked to help I had to think about the management of alcohol in a much more personal way. I was flummoxed and asked for help.

Part of that help came from an unexpected source which included the private sector. They very kindly forwarded me some of their written material including "How to Enjoy Life Without Alcohol" and "How to Motivate Someone to Seek Help to Give Up Drinking". They came from dryoutnow.com and were written by Dr Bruce Trathen, Consultant in Addiction Psychiatry. They were first published in 2008 by Triage Healthcare. I found this information singularly helpful in its clarity simplicity and honesty. I liked in particular the way it was constructed, inviting the person to first clarify whether or not they were physically addicted to alcohol, whether they planned to stop drinking completely or to continue drinking within healthy limits and more particularly whether or not they were ready to do something about it. The last chapter 'Are You Ready to Act Now?' posed and discussed ten very clear questions:

1. Have you made a completely honest commitment to yourself to totally cease all alcohol use for at least a period of months after detox?

2. Are you prepared to suffer disturbed sleep, feelings of agitation and to resist sometimes overwhelming cravings for alcohol for many months after your detox?

3. Are you prepared to keep on working at staying dry, drinking at safe limits for the rest of your life?

4. Do you honestly believe the gains you will make by ceasing alcohol use by far out way the losses?

5. Are you absolutely 100% convinced your overall quality of life will be improved by stopping drinking?

6. Are you aware that for the rest of your life you will remain at high risk of relapsing to damaging levels of alcohol consumption within a matter of days after taking your first drink?

7. Are you prepared to be on guard for the rest of your life against the little voice that will enter your head when most unexpected saying: "Go on – just one drink can't hurt – how could it?"

8. Are you prepared to do whatever it takes to stay off alcohol (or control it) in the long-term and give this absolute priority over everything else in your life?

9. Are you planning to stop drinking because you want to do this for yourself, and not solely for the benefit of another person?

10. Do you take full, personal responsibility for all the problems in your life, whether or not you believe they are caused by drinking?

They conclude that chapter with the following:

"You have now reached then end of this chapter and should be able to answer the question: Are you ready to act now?"

As I write this I am reminded of Tom who you met in one of the earlier chapters. He had not had any leave for two months when he first arrived and was slowly progressing through both escorted and unescorted leave. One day however, he decided to catch the bus down west to see a friend, to have a couple of drinks. When he was returned by the police I asked him whether he had paid for the alcohol this time. He smiled and said "Yes, £2.99." I was gobsmacked you could buy a bottle of vodka for that price. I think I pay more for milk! Anyway we continued the discussion and I asked him whether he felt alcohol was a problem. He said yes and no. Yes because the police had been involved but quite frankly, he couldn't see what the fuss was all about. I let him know his leave would be cancelled for 48 hours which he knew would happen. I then decided to ask him, although the decision had been made in relation to this incident, what action or consequence he would prefer on subsequent occasions? I think this is the direction we might continue to head in, namely inviting the men to think about what would be a reasonable consequence. We have tried this with a couple of the other men, when they breached leave conditions for various reasons. It seems to work okay, at least on a good day!

Alcohol abuse is still 'a work in progress' and it is probably still a bit haphazard. In some ways things have changed. When Dan first came to the unit he was adamant he was off both drugs and alcohol, and with naltrexone, had no cravings. He didn't believe alcohol would be a problem and so he wasn't interested in pharmacological support to maintain sobriety or developing a 'Plan B'. Owen similarly adopted an idealised position where alcohol would never be a problem. It was Vanessa, in a Reflective Practice Group, who remarked how it might have been too difficult to think about anything other than 'everything is all good' and to consider 'the bad parts' we all share.

Drugs

By the time our men arrive they have been detoxified often from extraordinary and varied amounts of any conceivable mind altering substances, which they have taken from an early age and for protracted periods of time. Recently one of our men, who was desperate for an experience ate the contents of his underarm roll-on deodorant. I don't know the physiology but have noted on various MRI, SPECT or CT head scan reports the phrase, 'appearances are consistent with polysubstance misuse'.

How difficult must it be for cognitively impaired people to 'remain mindful' of the adverse effects and consequences, to use judgement or be capable of personal responsibility.

Our principles are not dissimilar to how we have managed alcohol with random testing, suspension of leave and referral to Cornwall Drug and Alcohol Team (CDAT) for specialist advice. It was only when Dan was able to shift his position from "There is no problem doctor. I'll never touch drugs again" to one in which he was able to say he would use again, within two weeks of leaving hospital because he still misses that 'high'.

Wow! Now we had an opportunity to develop 'a plan B'. At least it afforded us the opportunity of beginning to think about contingencies and what might be needed. Dan had already done considerable work over 30 sessions with the psychologist when he had been in medium security. Together we were able to piece together something which might protect him. It included continuing the one hour weekly contact with Cornwall

Drug and Alcohol Team (CDAT) in the community to maintain his focus and commitment. This is life-long work but continuity with the same clinician is difficult to provide in a service with changing staff. We were also mindful, given the losses he had already experienced: losing his girlfriend, losing his home, losing his family, losing his financial independence and his repeated imprisonments, that losing escorted or unescorted leave was trivial in comparison. The other difficulty was trying to imagine what we were asking him to give up, particularly the 'highs'. The closest I came, was giving up sex. I asked Dan about this. He agreed with my comparison. Interestingly when I asked him which was better, he chose sex, and he described the intimacy and the closeness of the human touch. Dan has rekindled a relationship with his old girlfriend. He is being cherished and nourished for who he is as a person and so in turn is beginning to value himself. Maybe now there will be a sustainable shift.

Throughout the struggle with what is obvious, intoxication, threat and deception, there is a sadness.

The following poem was written by a man, with drug additions, who has since died. He left it with his Consultant to share with others.

Orphans

Light, sound, breath, pain
No mother's breast
No father's touch
Unwilling
Unwanted
Alone
Tiny hands close
On air
But have nothing
To cling to
For love
No brother's pride
No sister's cry
No Aunts or Uncles
Dropping by
For crying eyes
No lullabies
No joy, no toys
No bells to ring
In all the world
No sadder thing
Forget the womb
From which we're torn
Best not remember
Being born

Ian Goral (June '99)

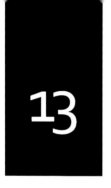

13 Personality disorders

"To hospitalise an antisocial patient usually leads to regret. His disruptive behaviour may grossly interfere with the treatment of other patients and may bring all therapeutic programmes to a grinding halt. Those patients will steal from, sexually exploit and assault other patients; they will also lie to and ridicule staff members, smuggle drugs and alcohol into the unit, ridicule the treatment philosophy and corrupt staff members into dishonest and unethical behaviours. Some will systematically destroy any therapeutic relationship other patients have developed with the treatment staff"

Gabbard, 2000 (thanks to Toby Mackinnon who emailed this to us from his talk).

Antisocial personality disorder

We weren't sure about writing a section about people with personality disorder and believe it's quite difficult to have a mixed unit. Certainly from our experience of visiting other units, similar observations are made. One of the problems is, people with a personality disorder require a different orientation than people with schizophrenia. The two groups don't always mix easily. While we understand the financial implications and economies of size, we believe if there is a genuine interest in wishing to work with people with personality disorders then this requires a dedicated response.

Certainly the experience of the team with Peter's continued behaviour over 15 months was one of exhaustion. Appropriately he was referred out of county. We did want to include a brief note however, because of the two pieces we read about anti-social personality disorder. The first is in a book by Meloy which a colleague lent me. The chapter on psychotherapy (pages 309 - 340) was particularly helpful. Here's the first sentences:

"The psychopathic process is not immune to psychotherapy, but it does present major counter transference and resistance issues to the mental health professional. The response of most clinicians to the psychopathic patient is to question the possibility of psychotherapeutic change, which may be either a counter transference reaction to psychopathic devaluation or a realistic decision based upon sound clinical judgement".

What Meloy then goes on to describe is issues to do with evaluation, treatability and severity. It is clear there are individuals who are so psychopathically disturbed that, in his opinion, no attempts should be made to treat them. He adds however, the decision to not treat should be made as carefully as the decision to offer treatment but often the sources of data are much more limited. He lists the following:

1. Sadistic aggressive behaviour in the patient's history that resulted in serious injury, maiming or death to the victim.
2. Complete absence of any remorse, justification or rationalisation for such behaviour.
3. Intelligence greater than or less than two standard deviations from the mean. This places the individual in the very superior or mildly mentally retarded range of general intelligence.
4. A historical absence of any capacity, or inclination, to form a bond or an emotional attachment to another person.
5. An apathistic fear of predation felt by experienced clinicians when in the patient's presence without any overt behaviour precipitating such a counter transference reaction.

Having had it refreshingly, but honestly, stated there are

occasions in which 'any' form of treatment is contra-indicated, was useful. It enabled us, to then read his section on counter transference. He included the therapeutic illusion, the illusionary treatment alliance, the fear of assault or harm, denial and deception; with denial being the most ubiquitous defence against anxiety generated by a violent patient. He also added helplessness, guilt, devaluation and loss of professional identity, hatred, the wish to destroy and the assumption of psychological complexity as additional means by which we become seduced and thrown off balance from doing the recovery work. He also described the predictable resistances which occur during psychotherapy including manipulative cycling, deceptive practice, malignant pseudo-identification and sadistic control.

The second piece is Larry Strasburger's article entitled 'The Treatment of Antisocial Syndromes: The Therapist's Feelings' which again explores the difficulties in working with this group. We don't think it's possible to do the work without coming to terms, and at times repeatedly having to come to terms with these aspects of this.

Before finishing this section, we would also like to add two other quotations on treating people with anti-social personality disorder.

"Patients may be labelled as untreatable with no recognition that it is the limits of our knowledge and ways of working which results in failure".

and

> "In my view such work requires an ability to stay with very difficult experiences and material and struggle to foster an understanding in working through very complex damaged aspects of a personality. It also requires an ability to struggle to maintain a dialogue with those who may long since have lost any belief that they can be understood or that their lives can be different. But then perhaps neither the public nor the courts really want to grapple with the problems which mentally disordered offenders (MDOs) present. It involves after all wrestling with what can go wrong with the human mind – and therefore with what can go wrong with all of us".

We don't have what it takes to work with people who have anti-social personality disorder. We have offered these contributions in good faith for others.

I'm not sure he has schizophrenia

We weren't quite sure where to insert this section but decided to put it in here, because anti-social personality disorder was the most likely diagnosis for Owen. The problem was we had already met him and he was well liked, didn't cause any trouble with the other men (who were obviously unwell) and just got on with it while he waited for the Ministry of Justice to discharge him.

Owen had come down from a medium secure unit. Although originally thought of as having an anti-social personality disorder, things didn't quite fit and his psychopathy check list score wasn't particularly high. There were some indications which led psychiatrists to wonder whether or not he might have schizophrenia. He was afforded a trial of medication and improved.

When we first met Owen he was medicated. He had been well for some months prior to transfer and continued to be so on our unit. In preparing a report, in which his continued detention needed to be justified, it became difficult to articulate the phenomena upon which the original diagnosis of schizophrenia had been made. It was a phrase which rang warning bells 'typical delusional beliefs' – without specifying what those beliefs might have been. Owen's own account was equally vague. 'Violent thoughts, becoming paranoid, people against me', but little else. I elected to defer to my colleagues who had seen him when unwell. We asked for a continuation of his section, which was granted. He remained the model patient and was eventually given a conditional discharge to the community, with follow-up from the community forensic team - this included an exclusion zone (an area Owen was not permitted to visit), employment and prohibition of drugs and alcohol.

Within perhaps a couple of months, Owen had drank, and while intoxicated, retaliated after he was punched by a passer-by. He was arrested, but as he had just been seen by the Community Forensic Team and deemed to be mentally well, he was not recalled to the psychiatric system. This was a sound decision by the Ministry of Justice. Instead he was electronically tagged and bailed. While waiting for his court appearance, Owen felt overwhelmed by the stress. He drank again and in the context of 'paranoia' and 'people looking at me' was recalled to hospital. We saw him again. He was almost the same, in that he was pleasant, polite, willing to please and be the model patient. The same person he had been, when with us for several months prior to his conditional discharge. However, and presumably in response to a particular line of questioning at the time, that I find difficult to recall, I briefly sensed Owen was someone who could be quite violent.

The dilemma I had was that once again I didn't feel he had schizophrenia. Two very experienced forensic colleagues felt differently. As he was due to appear in court in one week's time, Owen said how proud he was. He had met a girl, she was perfect and they were expecting their first child. Owen had described the prison hospital to me, where he essentially stayed in his cell for 23 hours a day, coming out only for meals and often being kept awake by other patients who were banging on their doors throughout the night. He was pleased to be back with us on a safe and homely unit. The problem however was what to present at the tribunal. If we felt he didn't have schizophrenia Owen might return to prison. This would potentially 'harden him'. The flipside was to ask the tribunal to consider this young man as having a future with his new and proud role as a parent and the long-standing support of his parents. However, could this 'excuse his behaviour'. We discussed the various pros and cons, including the integrity of the expert opinion for a tribunal and of hiding behind the clinician's role. We took the view that irrespective of diagnosis, Owen clearly had difficulties. Whether they were due to a pathological process or not, he could benefit from the skill and experience the clinical team might be able to offer in terms of providing a supervised structure and containment, both on the unit and as he left to return to the community.

As is so often the case, once the positions had been defined and the clinical material presented, people somehow feel more relaxed and open to different view points. It was Michaela who went back to thinking about the philosophy of the unit - Whole Life, individualised care and normalisation within our local community. Had we too become seduced by his pleasant nature and wanted to protect him from the consequences we would all normally face as members of the community? In the long run this would be a dis-service to Owen. Whilst we were happy to work with and support him, it was again the direct, open and honest clarity Michaela was able to model which enabled us to make a decision. Not easy but maybe, that was what the fear was about. I hadn't seen it first time round, denial being the most ubiquitous response to anxiety generated by a violent patient.

Borderline Personality Disorder

I have found working with people with Borderline Personality Disorder interesting. What remains the most useful approach for me is Dawson & McMillan's very readable book in Relationship Management. Here are some introductory sections:

> Sometime in my first year of residency the nurse woke me at 2 am to ask if I would help them with a young woman who had run off the ward. We found her banging her head against a wall. I knelt beside her and tried to convince her that what she was doing was unhelpful, mustering as much empathy, patience and positive regard as one can at that hour. She ignored my entreaty and continued, the nurses becoming impatient with both the woman and myself. I began to consider forcible removal and intramuscular medication. On the same ward another young woman, attractive in appearance and appearing neither severely depressed or psychotic, was receiving intensive psychotherapy. One evening she sliced open the right side of her neck with a razor blade, narrowly missing her carotid artery. She was put on heavier medication and closer observation. In the next few days we tiptoed around her asking ourselves if she were perhaps more depressed or psychotic than she appeared. Another young woman who had been

molested by her father was re-admitted for the seventh time following her numerous escapades with men of all ages and persuasions, illicit drug use and multiple overdoses. She was on a hunger strike having been placed in seclusion after she had broken windows and cut herself.

In Dawson and McMillan's introduction, a series of familiar clinical scenarios are described. They note that with the risk of suicide, the response has been to diagnose a disorder which serves the additional function of legitimising, if need be, compulsory treatment. The experience from this approach up to the early 1990s had been one of therapeutic nihilism and antipathy. Dawson and McMillan adopted a different stance. In particular they were intrigued by how this same group of people responded differently depending on how they were approached. They described a young man who was addicted to drugs and, when those drugs were refused, threatened to jump off a nearby bridge. They recognised the dilemma, namely that in the long-run hospitalisation would be unhelpful but should he jump, there would be an inquest where they would have to explain to their Head of Department, the administration, the coroner and in their imagination, a newspaper reporter as to why they had not hospitalised a man so sick and desperate.

Instead the authors began a discussion with the man: 'I don't want you to kill yourself, but I have no way of stopping you if that is truly what you wish to do. It is up to you. However I will continue to see you regularly'. Their view, articulated in their chapter entitled 'The Necessary Conceptual Leap' is that patients seek self definition and a resolution of their conflicts and discomfort by their externalised, interpersonal negotiation with others. They note how the patient's presentation as helpless and incompetent elicits the already controlling, definition-imposing authority of healthcare institutions which makes them feel more helpless and incompetent. The patient then tries to overcome this by gaining control of the situation using what they sense is the only currency at their disposal. They also note there is a special kind of control over others which comes from not being in control of one's self. "There is a special kind of self esteem and sense of power that must arise from being so chronically incompetent, hopeless and helpless, that one antagonises and defeats the best and brightest healthcare professionals." Recognising responses are socially constructed, they argue while we may not be able to change the person with borderline personality disorder, what we are able to change is our response to their presentation. Their relationship management is based on the premise that the person with borderline personality disorder is a responsible and competent adult. Although often hidden, this approach has also underscored Linehan's work: "... placing primary responsibility upon the patient to change her own life entails risks - literally of life or death - that the therapist must accept if treatment is to be successful. If the therapist cannot accept such a risk and strives to keep the patient alive at all costs, a patient will inevitably fail to achieve the goal of a life worth living. Acceptance of the possibility that the patient may commit suicide is an essential requisite..."

The difficulty is that my experience has almost exclusively been in the community and so I have little to offer in the inpatient setting of a low secure unit. I've included a copy of a letter we wrote to a journal, Australasian Psychiatry, in 2009 in order to see what is possible. It is reprinted with permission.

What is possible...
"Dear Sir

"Nothing happens until the doctor is touched by the patient" Jaspers, 1900.

We wish to describe the changes in response of a mental health service to deliberate self-harm (DSH). In 1993, the former Grampian's Psychiatric Services (GPS) was confronted with the increasingly difficult task of managing people with deliberate self-harm. Five single women with a mean average of 26.6 years and who met an average of 8.4 of nine DSM-IV criteria for borderline personality disorder were identified. On average, they had previously received 5.6 different diagnoses, had been admitted voluntarily on 12.5 occasions to 6.4 different hospitals but had become involuntary

186

within 6.4 days, with threats to leave or of further deliberate self-harm. They had been hospitalised for a mean total of 1015 days, had 1162 hours of seclusion and had received a mean of 14 different psychotropic agents. Four had received electro-convulsive therapy (ECT). All had significant medical histories including meningitis, cardiac murmurs, deep vein thrombosis, pelvic inflammatory disease and Hepatitis C. All had been sexually abused from a mean age of 7.25 years, three had comorbid substance abuse and four had a forensic history. Deliberate self-harm included threatened or actual immolation, mutilation of genitals, ingestion of foreign bodies, jumping from buildings or walking in front of cars and trains. Threats to staff were personal, with a forensic history including arson, siege, threats to kill, stalking and armed robbery. Two patients had been imprisoned.

To put these figures in context, GPS was one of 22 Victorian Area Mental Health Services and had a population of 204,208 spread across 48,112 square kilometres. There was 10.6% unemployment, 16% of families were 'single parents' and 20% of households received less than £12,000 per annum. Available resources included a fixed workforce derived from two large regional asylums in the process of closure, a planned 40% budget reduction over two years and six psychiatrists. The political backdrop included local, multi-agency concern, a focus on psychotic disorders and de-institutionalisation, and a trend towards police shootings.

In 1994, GPS began an organisational, community-based model of care, which resulted in these same five women receiving a different service. GPS - initiated phone calls increased from 2.5 to 79.5, home visits from 4.0 to 151.3 and crisis contacts from 0.8 to 17 per person. The mean number of admissions, length of stay and time in seclusion fell to 7, 103.2 days and 21.6 hours respectively. The mean number of psychotropic medication dropped to 2.8 per person with one receiving ECT. Following the use of this model, no new patient became as severely disturbed as these five women had become.

For health-giving professionals, the development of a humane understanding of deliberate self-harm was regarded as central, GPS used the conceptual framework of abnormal illness behaviour whereby deliberate self-harm was seen as 'a calling card' by which people could make contact, at least with professionals who had a duty to respond. Management revolved around seeing a person regularly rather than in crisis – a "You don't need to harm yourself, I will see you anyway", social contact became uncoupled from deliberate self-harm. That is, people with deliberate self-harm were embraced rather than alienated as service users. Realistic expectations including an acknowledgment of the iatrogenic effects of protracted admissions and the inappropriate use of medication led to a model whereby people were neither admitted nor evicted onto the street. Rather, people could be cared for in a different way. While ultimately revised, the statement that hospital and medication were unhelpful gave clinicians permission to respond in a different way. The guidelines eventually included the flexibility of brief, up to 48-hour admission for diagnostic clarification or to defuse an exhausted community. Regular respite admission and a patient-based voucher system in which the patient chose when to use a predetermined number of inpatient days per year were also explored. No sustainable change was noted despite multiple psychotropic use. Also because of the potential for the medicalisation of psychosocial disadvantage and for acting out, a decision was made to not prescribe to new patients, and to gradually invite medication reduction in existing patients. For those patients who were unable to tolerate this offer, medication was kept constant. Crises were managed by two competent adults, the patient and the case manager. The task was to discover what had happened and what could be done differently with live problems from a community existence. Tiny changes were reinforced, like phoning before cutting which was acknowledged as a major achievement after weeks of work. Regular contact was a fundamental principle, each person in the relationship keeping the same time each week, with each developing an ability to contain their distress until the next appointment. A 'sliding scale of insulin' approach to exceptional need followed by return to regular contact allowed for flexibility. The diagnosis, risk and personal responsibility of suicide was discussed with the patient and, with consent, with other family members.

A specialist team was not established as it was thought that to do so may create the possibility of failure, should key individuals leave or become overwhelmed by the responsibility. Instead, each clinician became part of an intersecting network of service responses that together could support the person in the community. The patient was encouraged to develop a relationship with the service as a whole, as well as with a single case manager. Seconds were nominated and introduced for roster change, holidays and sick leave and for handover at pre-arranged times. Realistic caseloads were important.

A medico-legally safe environment within which staff could work in the community was discussed with management, hospital solicitors and subsequently the coroner. Having been appraised of the dilemmas, their support was both crucial and surprisingly forthcoming. Training over a 12 month period included a questionnaire and a one page summary of the model. These were distributed to the acute, community and inpatient components of the psychiatric service, the mainstreamed general hospital and to those agencies with whom the patient continued to have contact. The latter included the ambulance service, police, general practitioners and non-government agencies. Rather than requiring agencies to agree, the presentations focused on understanding how and why care was being delivered in a different way. In addition, a two day in-service was available for interested clinicians. The voluntary nature was an acknowledgment that, for some clinicians, deliberate self-harm was not their interest area. A workbook accompanied the course with four essential references addressing relationship management, medico-legal dilemmas, splitting and malignant alienation. Subsequently, a short practical text has been published that describes the development of specific management plans for each person which can be consistently administered across services and two useful papers on professional risk taking. These same principles of care were later introduced and accepted by the child and adolescent service.

Caring in a different way offered a clinical approach

and softened previous therapeutic nihilism and antipathy. There were difficulties including the practicalities of ensuring regular referral to readily available, consistently applied management plans and for the quiet patience of the confident clinician. For some, threats were too frightening and a conservatism remained. Managing this split was important, modelling as it does an ability to accept different opinions and to avoid polarisation. While successful in reducing hospitalisation and inappropriate prescribing, managing long-term dysphoria and clinician fatigue was underestimated.

For the service wishing to work with people with deliberate self-harm, morale is important. Peer support and review, prospectively collecting data with diagnostic clarity rather than pejorative labelling, and knowing the results of that data are important. Unique observations, the unexpected finding of significant medical histories unrelated to deliberate self-harm, the clinical triad of multiple diagnoses, multiple admissions and multiple medications as a diagnostic marker, and the differing length of stays between hospitals and psychiatrists were intriguing. Contact with specialist providers and access to journals and conferences also maintains enthusiasm."

John Little and Janice Rouhan

It is sad to see people with borderline personality disorder being incarcerated when it is possible to do it another way.

14 Acquired brain injury

The original idea of having a male low secure unit in Cornwall was to provide an opportunity for Cornish men, (who had either committed offences while mentally ill or, due to their challenging behaviour), currently managed out of county, to return to Cornwall. This meant they could be closer to their families and helped to reduce the financial implications of not having a local unit. As we began to develop confidence and started to successfully discharge people, we began to consider a broader population group. When a referral came in for a person who had an acquired brain injury, we were hesitant. Although I hadn't known him, Michaela had worked with him successfully in the community some years earlier. (He will be referred to as Graham). Graham had been repatriated from a two to three year period in an out of county, head injury unit. The referral letter had indicated quite a marked change and deterioration since that time. Feeling confident and capable, given our recent apparent successes, we wanted to offer him an opportunity to experience something of the Bowman Unit programme. We hadn't wanted to tune into the very faint warning bell.

The man was nearly 40 and his head injury was acquired almost 20 years earlier. In the descriptions it seemed somewhat trivial. He had experienced a closed head injury with only 'a few seconds' loss of consciousness. He had also received a significant financial compensation package. While at one point we did consider whether or not there was an element of abnormal illness behaviour, subsequent clinical testing confirmed significant problems in his ability to organise and carry out tasks which required sequencing and planning. By way of example, and because he was both unable and unwilling to sit with formal testing, our psychologist described the following account of his escorted visit to the supermarket.

"This real world assessment took the form of asking him to both plan and cook a meal from scratch with minimal support. Firstly, when shopping for the ingredients he showed relatively poor sequencing skills, typically associated with executive functioning. This poor sequencing and planning was demonstrated by the following: (1) leaving without a shopping list; (2) walking past all the trolleys and baskets then having to go back for them when his arms and hands were full; (3) returning to the same aisle several times rather than picking up two separate items stored next to each other on the same trip; (4) becoming side-tracked by tonic water and (5) after having all items scanned at the checkout, realising he didn't have enough money to pay for them."

He had come to us from the community. They were at their wits end on how best to continue to manage his reckless driving, inappropriate sexual relationships with vulnerable females, physical destructiveness of property alongside his rapid and threatening verbal violence when his immediate requests were not met. Unable to manage on the general adult unit, he was transferred to the psychiatric intensive care unit (PICU) where swift responses to boundary violations were an important and appropriate part of their culture and function. They too had expressed difficulties in ensuring a sustained improvement and accordingly referred him to us for consideration. The hope was that a longer period of containment and management might effect a robust and sustainable change in his behaviour.

Initially he was verbally and physically violent. He broke doors, absconded and made sexually inappropriate comments and malicious and unfounded allegations towards staff. If true, these would have cost those staff their jobs. Staff became frustrated, exhausted and angry as he would later tearfully retract those same allegations saying he had wanted to get back at a staff member for not meeting his immediate demands. We tried understanding the various losses he had experienced recently both personally and generally in terms of his loss of freedom. He said his present existence was not a life, he didn't want to be in hospital, he didn't want to be on medication and all he wanted was to be able to leave hospital, have a girlfriend and live normally. Frustration and anger quickly spilled over with broken doors and the whole window being kicked out of its frame so the integrity and security of the unit was jeopardised. Loss of leave compounded the frustration as no sooner had he been given a period of leave then a further angry outburst resulted in a further loss of his leave. Increasingly, both he and the team got backed into a corner from which there appeared no easy resolution.

He complained he wasn't able to manage his anger for the periods of time we were asking him to because "I have a brain injury." We tried sitting with him, discussing our dilemmas and inviting him to put together a plan which might work. Again initially it seemed as if he appreciated being spoken to as an responsible adult, but again without a sustainable change. We tried positively reinforcing small changes. We sat with him as we began to develop what seemed to us to be a readily achievable activity plan over the weekend with the prospect of leave on the Monday. The targets were deliberately set low and included those activities he would ordinarily be doing. These included a tidy room which he usually maintained, watering his plants which he routinely did as he had a keen interest and ability in the garden. While he was able to manage, the delay from Sunday to Monday was too long and once again he became volatile on the Sunday evening and lost his leave. We acknowledged that maybe we had left the gap between task completion and leave too long. We were also mindful of the possibility he may genuinely not have been able to manage his frustration. The activities, the delay and what we were expecting of him was in fact cognitively too difficult for him. We tried 'random acts of kindness' whereby we would note the smallest behaviour and then, without fuss, facilitate leave. By way of example, he was very much an outdoor man and found it very difficult being cooped up in a low secure unit. One morning he repeatedly approached the staff for some new toothpaste and interrupted the meeting we were in. We weren't able to do this immediately. We told him this but that we would by the end of the shift. On this occasion he was able to walk away without retaliatory violence. Immediately after the meeting, we went up to him and said something along the lines of "Noticed how you coped with wanting the toothpaste without becoming angry. Would you like to go out for a walk?" Again improvements proved temporary.

We were somewhat at a loss. We felt we had failed and along with the various other stressors occurring on the unit at the time, were seduced into developing a policy for any breach. At reflective practice, I became aware we had just contributed to institutionalisation. I had children and at times it was difficult to balance each of their individual needs. On the unit, we now had 14 people to consider. In order to mange my anxiety I was tempted into controlling multiple and complex clinical demands by a one size fits all approach. It was again Michaela who addressed this retreat into an institutionalised response. She reminded us of our commitment to an individualised, specific programme for each person. Michaela made it simple, unequivocal and fair. The chap understood, we understood and we could be consistent across shifts. Everyone who needed it, had a copy of his care plan.

One of the reasons we wanted to include this example was to describe the process of change which occurred on the unit as an adaptation to a new and unfamiliar clinical presentation - acquired brain injuries.

We were deliberately slow in writing this chapter and even uncertain as to whether we should include it. There is an obvious temptation, particularly when finances are stretched, to accommodate all possible patients who may benefit from a low secure setting without thinking about the impact on the effectiveness of the overall unit. To include this chapter also might suggest or advertise we can mange people with acquired brain injuries. We were able to clarify that long standing, static injuries remain static. An admission to a low secure unit provided an opportunity, confirmed the permanence of a long standing brain injury and suggested for this man a long-term, out of county, residential care placement was required. There are costs however and with this particular chap, costs to the fabric of a building and to the personal safety of the staff and the other men. The costs also included an impact on the morale of the unit and its underlying philosophy. There seemed to be a shift from a person-centred approach towards a behavioural programme. The clinical balance required struggling with containment, which could have easily become too tight and freedom, which could equally easily become permissive.

Graham had been known to our service and had previously responded to a protracted admission to a specialist head injury unit. We were feeling confident and wanted to offer him a chance. However, we're not sure we would offer a placement to another person with an acquired brain injury in the future. We could now hear that warning bell ringing!

five

The long haul...

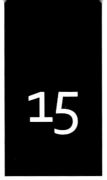

15 | Losing focus

In this section we wanted to describe some of the experiences and thoughts we struggle with when care is long-term.

We feel it is better to talk about rather than hide these everyday feelings. We then have a chance of managing them differently rather than continuing to complain and let our angry feelings emerge in unhelpful ways. Accordingly, the issues that arise are a way of beginning to collect together clinical experience, to reconnect with the art, rather than just the science of psychiatry. Again, I think it is the non-medical staff who do this well, and do so without necessarily being aware of how skilled and experienced they are at managing matters which arise within chronic containment.

Prior to starting on Bowman and in addition to the fear I experienced, I also wondered whether or not progress may be too slow for my taste. Whether I would become overwhelmed by the seemingly hopeless futility of chronic care. I was reminded of playing snooker. Dad introduced us to this wonderful game. For anyone who is familiar with it, you will be aware of sometimes losing focus. All you seem to be doing is hitting the balls around the table without being able to pot any of them. It seems there is a lull in the game. It requires an energy and ability to regain focus, to concentrate and continue onwards. Being watchful for the little things which may be easily overlooked. This reminded me of Tom. All we seemed to be doing, was nagging and nagging to get him to shower. Then one day Tom came up and asked in his characteristic style, "Is the music on today Miss?" Brilliant!

Gingerbread men

I had a job in an eel factory and loved it. On the first day, you had to hop into a tank of live eels and remove the dead ones. As a student, three months holiday was the only time when you could make enough money for the rest of the year so I just got on with it. Occasionally there was overtime available and as students we would leap at the chance. I asked one of the other men at the factory why they didn't volunteer. He was clear and adamant. He worked from nine to five Monday to Friday and no more. I was taken aback, I had expected people would be as interested in and needing the money as much as I did.

I had a similar experience recently. The team had been trying to work with Dean, a young man who despite our best efforts remained partially treated. We were trying to engage him in activities and he would get increasingly cross with us, saying he wasn't interested in anything. As I was talking to him I remembered similar comments being made to me when I was growing up. "John, you should have a hobby. You should broaden your interests. You should get involved in music. You should do this, that and the next thing." I was quite happy being and doing nothing so Dean and I were able to reach some common ground. Perhaps more precisely, I was able to accept and acknowledge where he was coming from. For Dean, life was about trying to leave hospital, live a normal life, and for him, a normal life was sitting at home, not working, occasionally going out and doing some shopping, but that was it. If an activity happened to come along which interested him then so be it, but he felt no inclination or interest in doing anything else.

It was quite useful for me to read the section on 'The Gingerbread Man' in a book to do with disappointment. The suggestion was there is a temptation to make "gingerbread cut-outs" of all of us, that we should all be the same, with the same aspirations. Sometimes it's not the case. Sometimes though, it can also be an excuse for giving up. In particular, I wondered whether or not I had been manoeuvred into feelings of hopelessness, of giving up and of acquiescing, perhaps like his mum felt. On further reflection we were able to see perhaps, we had allowed ourselves to become defeated as Dean may also have become. Everyone had given up.

Institutionalisation

It's a funny old thing institutionalisation. I was nervous about whether I would fit in when I first arrived but people made me feel welcome. I slowly began to find my way around, see how things worked, to get to know the staff and they got to know me. I fell into a routine of seeing each of the men on Monday, the unit round on Tuesday and in the afternoon the HCR-20 (a risk assessment tool) or care plans and continuing professional development on Wednesday. Tribunals, report writing, family meetings and out of county assessments were on Thursdays and Fridays. I too had become institutionalised.

Will told me that for six years he had been part of a UK rapid reaction force, attached to 3-Commando Brigade who, within a 24 to 48 hour period, could be deployed anywhere in the world. What struck me, was his observation that when he left, along with his colleagues who had also left, Will found it extraordinarily difficult to settle to one job. Although as you might imagine they were very able men and women, it seemed they too had found it difficult to adjust and adapt to a regular routine. They had become institutionalised. I asked how long it took them to settle. He said three years. Six years of becoming attached to one environment, three years to become de-institutionalised and this was with a competent, able and actively functioning member of the community. Some of our men had progressed down through high, medium and low secure hospitals over 17, 21 and 33 years. In terms of outcomes, the clinically relevant measure seemed to be whether or not they were able to move to the next step.

Dependency

Becky describes another important issue when working in a slow stream rehabilitation unit:

Acceptance

Trying to imagine my life without family, friends, and work is near impossible. This is reality for many of the men on our unit, so it may not be surprising that for some, the Bowman community is considered all they've got. For some of these men, we are their only network and provide the only relationships they have. This is unavoidable, though we endeavour to encourage and support healthy relationships with other people, this can prove difficult. Some become dependant on the support or simply the comfort of regular interactions. Some are desperate to be able to live independently but through fear avoid making this step, some even sabotage their exit plan consciously or subconsciously.

One man springs to mind. He has decided to put his past behind him, including all the people in it. He admitted (before leaving to live in the community) to feeling at times that he didn't want to leave even if only for the relationships he'd built with staff while on the unit. These relationships for him are as important, I presume, as the relationships I have with my friends and family. He had to leave and build his life from scratch. This is so daunting and a task I find very hard to even contemplate. He fears never being able to construct the kinds of relationships he forged during his stay on the unit again.

Professionally speaking, we may consider this unhealthy and more appropriate relationships should be sought and ordinarily they would be, but being in hospital, leaving hospital and having to start afresh isn't ordinary. We are human too, quite simply we also look for and need bonds. A bond is essential when expecting to support someone so it seems obvious to me that for some, this bond may want to remain.

When you think about it, who are the people in society most likely to understand, appreciate and accept those with mental health problems? Who in society are people with mental health problems most likely to appreciate and accept in their lives? I don't feel this should be taboo. However we need to be able to question the healthiness of a relationship and know where the boundaries lie.

Risk

Ian our new psychologist, made an interesting comment. In essence he said if we believe we are doing everything right, we're probably doing something wrong. It made me think about being uncertain. The low secure unit population is distinctive and as yet there isn't literature which can guide us. Our men are likely to be excluded from easily conducted, randomised control research because of the complexity of their presentation. As such we rely on our clinical experience, on extrapolating from that experience, and from feeling our way. It's as if we are on a tightrope. Carefully and cautiously we are trying to cross, but the other side is not easily visible. As we inch our way across, it requires a quiet confidence to maintain balance amidst the winds of self doubt and criticism. We may need to pause and re-steady ourselves before progressing. We may become overwhelmed and paralysed and ultimately unable to move any of our men. At times the risks feel personal. It's reassuring being part of a team.

Knights in shining armour

Why is it as healthcare professionals, we want to care for those less fortunate than ourselves? Is it because we are caring individuals or is it because helping others makes us feel better about ourselves? Or is it a bit of both? If so, what happens when we can't help someone?

As healthcare professionals working on Bowman Unit our aim is to help the men who stay with us. When we are successful and see our men move forward we usually feel happy for them as well as feeling happy with ourselves for a job well done. To some extent we are motivated by a desire to help or rescue others.

However, when we confront a situation and don't know how to help, the tables are turned. We may become motivated by a desire to remove the feelings of guilt, fear or impotency which result from being at the limits of our knowledge and expertise.

It wasn't until recently the team enabled me to see I may be contributing to a problem. Dean had largely remained unchanged since his arrival on Bowman Unit and had repeatedly misused his leave. I was aware I had been sitting with him and trying to find and offer, yet another opportunity for him to have leave as he argued he would no longer abscond or drink while away. I was also aware that on most occasions when we met he was becoming increasingly angry with me.

The team enabled me to see that I too had become involved in what was akin to an abusive domestic relationship: presumably similar to the one he had with his mother. Dean would become angry and insistent with his demands and then became, if not pleasant, no longer angry when they were to some extent met. Our psychologist, Ian was able to identify this as a potential negative reinforcement schedule. We felt guilty at not being able help Dean as much as we would like and his aggression compounded this. Our guilt at not being able to make him better was facilitating a loss of objectivity. We were starting to make decisions to make us feel better. Decreasing our discomfort and calming Dean was also reinforcing as it is difficult to let someone down. It could have been our son or our brother. Our denial, or more particularly my denial of my own impotency and the sadness at the reality of Dean's situation was too uncomfortable, and I had retreated to the rescuing role.

As a result, I slowly began to change my approach. I sought the support of the team as I was finding it difficult. At times though, I felt I was in a space where I was grounded and clear, when I could say to Dean we were at the limits of our expertise. We were clear about the expectations we had of him in terms of the activities he had to do prior to getting leave. We could suggest he return to unescorted leave in a graduated and sequential way and it was clearly mapped out for all. Having returned to an adult role, things began to become easier and Dean was able to make more constructive use of his plan.

Working in the field of mental health can be a tricky old thing at times.

Feeling a fraud

It's a funny thing self doubt. You wonder when 'real forensic patients' arrive whether everyone will discover that you believe you are a fraud and the pack of cards will come tumbling down. I discussed this recently with two of my colleagues, Michaela and Iain. They acknowledged similar thoughts from time to time but were also clear while we may not be specifically trained, what we do bring is ourselves and a willingness to reveal that part of ourselves. As part of that, we keep busy, always looking for the next achievement which is both exciting but ultimately exhausting. They reminded me I could safely be part of a team. I could begin to see beyond a traditional style of practice which had emphasised clinical autonomy and individual responsibility.

16 Anger

The sheer frustration of it all

I think we've all made this complaint from time to time, namely, the work is difficult enough without unnecessary paperwork and duplication of activity. Form filling, manager's reviews and then the duplicated first tier tribunals. Having to beg for money for any of the activities we might wish to undertake with our men. To repeatedly justify each and every request, even though the arguments remain the same. For leaders like Michaela 'the fact of the matter is, organisations such as schools and hospitals, like dragons, eat hero innovators for breakfast'. As someone said recently "it's not what I came into this job for, I wanted to work with people."

It's not fair

This is an interesting observation that Becky made:

The right way

I strive to live my life the 'right' way for fear of consequences and/or because I'm morally obliged. Then there are those who live their life carelessly, with no regard for laws or ethics and appear to get away with it. Some of those end up on our doorstep and at times like other members of the public I find myself questioning how's this fair?

How has it come to be that some people abuse drugs, commit crimes and hurt the people around them and end up in a hospital where they are accommodated, fed, treated and supported 24/7? This is a simplistic view but one I cannot stop from fleetingly crossing my mind, I say fleetingly because I'm quickly reminded of this question: would I swap my life with theirs? Would I even want to spend a day in their life? The answer is no. I value these men and their experiences. They deserve to be proud of the remarkable human beings they are but I would never choose to go through what they've gone through to earn me a stay in a low secure hospital.

I highly rate the service we provide and if I needed to be supported by any psychiatric team it'd be ours but I would never ask to experience an enduring mental illness and be sectioned as a result. How fair is it that some people get dealt that card?

While further resentment may be fuelled by the benefit payments also received but I still wouldn't swap. One guy who spent some time on our unit used to jovially tease "you pay my benefits" and we'd reply "you earn me my wages!" It's just what makes the world go around. It may indeed be that the men on our unit need our professional skills to support them and if it wasn't for the mental illness they're experiencing we would need to find a job elsewhere."

Lone Worker

Mark is our occupational therapist (OT):

Mark

For me, the early days were characterised by feeling the pressure to perform in terms of producing positive results and outcomes to prove ones usefulness and value to the team as a whole. It is difficult to under-estimate the pressure I felt in terms of being one of a kind, meaning, I was the only occupational therapist, compared to an overwhelming number of registered mental nurses (RMNs) and healthcare assistants (HCAs). I recognise this situation was not exclusive to me and there are other professional groups in precisely the same situation. I point this out, because it is different from my previous community job where there was a more even spread of disciplines and a more generic style of working. As a lone representative of occupational therapy it also felt as though my part in the grand scheme of things is relatively insignificant.

Co-ordination of activities can be problematic as

it is not clear precisely who tasks can be delegated to. For example, nursing staff delegate nursing tasks to the healthcare assistants (HCAs) but there is no-one specifically available to work alongside me to run activities. There are occasions when planned activities happen simultaneously. While this may be beneficial in terms of offering choice, given we have a maximum of 14 patients, there could be times when patients miss out un-necessarily. The nursing staff's shift patterns make it difficult to reliably or consistently plan the joint running of activity groups.

An observation, which may seem obvious but which matters in relation to running regular time-tabled groups, is individual staff differences in terms of personality and interests are highly significant to the success or otherwise of groups and planned 1:1 activities. Simply allocating anyone who can be freed up from other duties will not yield the best result.

The shift patterns also lead to risk of the team splitting as the opposing shifts develop their own strategies for dealing with specific patients and their challenging behaviour which results in lack of consistency in following care plans. However, as the unit has evolved there has been a far greater degree of shared responsibility for the running of activities. Patients are fortunate to have access to a wide choice of activities on the unit and where appropriate in the community. healthcare assistants in particular, have been encouraged to run activities linked to their own leisure interests. One example being the music group which is both popular and successful.

Another issue I was aware of was the potential conflict arising from the varied range of roles and responsibilities within my job. For example, how much should I focus on social inclusion and the importance of providing opportunities to work with the men in community settings compared to providing activities on the unit? How much time to individual rather than group work? How much time should I give to setting up and running a general daily activity programme for the unit rather than one more specifically focussed on individual need? I had all these questions and while I could and did seek advice from others, ultimately (and of course that's what I'm paid to do) I had to make those decisions and take responsibility for them.

I can also fondly recall many events from this early period and middle period (although at the time some of these events were actually quite stressful). Trying in vain to gather the men together to participate in planned activity groups. Let's not forget these are individuals who are compromised in terms of experiencing on-going positive symptoms of psychosis as well as the negative symptoms such as lacking drive, initiative, motivation, poverty of ideas and whose experiences are often overlaid with anti-social personality traits, early life trauma, and institutionalisation. My attempts to gather people together for groups was made more difficult due to the lack of clarity as to whether I could rely on healthcare assistant (HCA) support staff to assist me given there are no dedicated occupational therapy (OT) support staff.

There were situations which were actually quite comical, such as frantically gathering people together and then losing them from the room while attempting to gather others who were less motivated to come - in order to encourage as many of the men as possible to participate.

I recall escorting one of the men to enable him to join in with a local community based horticulture project and observing the reaction of his peers when he chose to introduce himself with, "Hi, I'm Paul, I'm a psychopath."

Another memory is of escorting another of our men into Bodmin. Prior to leaving the unit I felt I had explained, the terms and conditions of his leave. Unfortunately, he chose to completely ignore the rules on buying lottery scratch cards. He took issue with being reminded this was not allowed. He then made it clear he wouldn't cooperate with the rest of the leave plan, leaving me with the option of following him hot-foot back to the unit as he angrily strode out at a walking pace which bordered on running!

On a different leave event, with another of the men, we were in town doing some clothes shopping when for some unexplained reason he became angry due to misconstruing an exchange between passing strangers. This left me with the delicate task of attempting to return him calmly to the unit while trying to keep additional stimulation to a minimum.

One of the men had a passion for steam trains. As there is a steam railway on a local branch line I was able to facilitate a monthly trip out on the train. Some folk just can't be hurried and this guy is certainly one of them. Virtually any method employed to hurry him along made absolutely no difference to his slow, methodical and slightly obsessional way of proceeding. In terms of arranging this activity, he would always want to smoke a cigarette at the half-way point on the train journey. Because of regulations about smoking in public, this involved having to leave the train and exit the property of the railway company via a pedestrian bridge. The stop-over period before the train was due to leave again was only about five minutes. Can you imagine the scene there would always be with only seconds to spare to get back on the train after a slow smoke and a slow amble back over the bridge? As far as he was concerned the train would just have to wait but of course I knew it had a timetable to keep to and had to use all my powers of persuasion and encouragement to ensure we were not left standing on an empty platform.

My knowledge of the interests of another of the men resulted in a referral to the local volunteer centre. The idea was for him to work behind the scenes in a local charity shop helping to prepare goods for sale. Setting this up required a considerable degree of delicate diplomacy and management due to his risk assessment profile. For a short period during which I escorted him there each week, this appeared to be successful. However, as his confidence grew, his ulterior and non-altruistic motive for participating became clearer. He is well known for his wheeling and dealing, being affectionately referred to as the "Del Boy of Bowman Unit". It slowly dawned on me he was using this as an opportunity to buy items from the back of the shop at discounted prices, which he was selling on to other patients for a profit! Once he had been rumbled, and once I understood his attachment to me meant he was unwilling to attend his work placement with a different member of staff the whole plan was clearly not sustainable.

In retelling these events, I am aware the reader is likely to form the impression these are examples of unsafe practices. However, all these events were carried out following team discussion and use of Section 17 leave plans. I suppose they stand as examples as to how we, as a team, have learnt from our experiences as we have gone along. While they could have potentially developed into more serious and risky situations they highlight the fact that the team are constantly striving to strike the right balance between risk assessment and management through a recovery focussed model of care.

As has been said in other chapters of the book, we don't always get things perfectly right but there is a positive willingness to co-operate, learn from our mistakes and to do our best which makes for an enjoyable and rewarding work environment. The Locum Psychiatrist at the time was keen that all patients should attend the unit based activity schedule and for this to be clearly recorded and measured. Leave and transfer to less secure settings should then be conditional upon regular attendance at these activities. The psychiatrist's view was that we should create a culture of expectation, patients should be self motivated to attend these groups without the need for prompting from staff. In my experience, if I were simply to run the activity without making the effort to gather people first, this would result in very few, if any of the men attending due to the degree of their difficulties with motivation and institutionalisation.

The past year has been characterised by a period of regrouping and consolidation. We have had the opportunity to take a fresh look at the culture, ethos and philosophy of the unit as a whole team. The current locum consultant psychiatrist's preferred working style is to foster a culture of autonomy, innovation and shared responsibility to encourage positive risk taking. As a result, we have been able to move on many of the original patients to less secure settings and have forged good links with other service providers within the organisation which work with our men in both hospital and community settings. Time will tell what will happen next.

If only they were all like me ...

It's a sensitive issue to talk about staff differences. In an earlier life I had become intrigued by the different length of stays different psychiatrists had for people with borderline personality disorder and wanted to examine this a little more closely. My professor at the time wouldn't be part of this study as he felt it ran the very real risk of blaming staff. I listened and accepted his refusal as well as his suggestion of trying to demonstrate the effectiveness of our treatment approach in another way. It wasn't until relatively recently I thought about this again in relation to two of the men on our unit who had a personality disorder. Complicated to manage, I also knew the principles of care we had developed over ten years had been successful. It seemed that if we were all able to consistently apply those same principles of relationship management, then we too could sustain effective management. After 30 plus years of institutional care this transpired to be overly optimistic. It had been helpful for the other young man who hadn't become so entrenched in the mental health system and was able to be returned to the community and offered a different experience. However, it did remind me of that old saying, 'if only everyone was like me ...' I can now see it's better that everyone isn't like me for all sorts of reasons, some of which I will share here.

I could see that seeking homogeneity in approach was actually a futile attempt at trying to manage my own discomfort when random, out of control events so easily sparked off yet another conflict. I could see having a heterogeneous staff group reflected the real world. We must all learn to manage people who we meet and appear to share little with except for the silhouette of a common humanity. I also could understand I hadn't allowed myself to appreciate or to consider what others bring to the clinical situation that I can't, and in so doing relate to people I had difficulty with. To see other people make real headway where I had been ineffective and impotent is in essence to be a team member. On a good day, (perhaps it doesn't happen as often as it might), I might well begin to wonder, explore and become curious as to how we click with some people and not with others. So the answer to the statement, "if only they were all like me ..." the answer is equally simple "thank goodness they're not!"

Anger comes in a variety of guises Maltsberger and Buie's article in the references, explores the various ways in which anger can sneak out and is worth a read.

17 Not just a B number

People, not pieces of paper

Taking a person's history into account is important when considering risk and the best ways to provide care for them. It allows us to make educated judgements. It is important, though, that we do not allow our knowledge of a person's illness and their past to get in the way when first meeting them. I feel it's important to greet new patients as if I know nothing about them, allowing me to be with them as I would with anyone else I meet and allowing them to present themselves as they wish to be perceived. For many new patients our rehabilitation and recovery unit is considered a fresh start, they hope to leave the past behind them and move on. Many of our men say they find it hard to move on when they feel people around them remind them of their past. They are very aware their notes and reports follow them everywhere they go, in fact, their notes tend to arrive before they do.

As already mentioned, a person's history is

227

important when assessing risk. We cannot afford to be flippant about past dangerous or violent thoughts and behaviour but if you are over cautious it's likely you'll come across as guarded and stand-offish; not an effective way to build a professional and trusting relationship. This is also likely to make the men feel pre-judged, ostracised and feel they cannot open to you. We mustn't be naive to risk and must always remain vigilant but this can be discreet and/or managed with 'physical', 'relational' and 'procedural' security where set standards are put in place to maintain safety. It's often best, though, when questioned why there is need for caution to be honest and explain the reasons rather than making vague excuses.

When I first started working on this unit, I had no experience in mental health, psychiatric units or locked environments. I was anxious, not just because it was unfamiliar to me but also because of so-called 'scare-mongering'. The majority of staff had much experience in these environments and many had worked with some of the patients we were expecting to arrive at the unit. Naturally there was lots of discussion, exchanging of knowledge and experience, and although certainly not deliberately so, it incited some fear in me. Not just a fear of the unknown now, a fear of what was known. From reading the mens' notes before they arrived, taking note of the list of incidents they may have been involved

228

in, it was easy to assume I ought to expect some frightening behaviour. What I have since learned is that in the majority of cases these behaviours were demonstrated in their past. While we should always remain concerned about dangerous behaviour that concern is less relevant today and should not get in the way of us treating our men as we'd wish to be treated.

Another impression, easy to make from reading notes and the substantial records of odd and bizarre behaviour is that some men are so unwell you cannot imagine them functioning in any typically 'human' manner. It may seem surprising it is possible to relate to our men. We can engage with them in very 'normal' ways. I've been asked by friends if it's possible to have conversations with the men on our unit; of course it is! Many interactions are no different to those I'd have with people in the community. Indeed some are odd and contain delusional and bizarre ideas, but with everyone on the unit it is possible to relate with them in some way. Some you would not be able to pick out, and tell they experience mental health problems, from a room of people picked randomly from the community.

The way I relate to the men on the unit is no different to the way in which I relate to my colleagues and friends. There are just different boundaries and expectations on the professional relationship. So although it's necessary to read notes and be aware of risk, it's important to allow yourself to be open-minded enough to allow your original perception to be challenged at times. Our patients are people, not pieces of paper and are very likely to squash your first judgement of them once you get to know them.

When we start working with the men, spending hours of each day with them, you start to see each person as 'a whole'; their unique personality, particular traits and quirks, what they are capable of, their drive, their likes and dislikes, their interactions with family and friends. You also see how different each person's illness is in contrast to how definite the titles of Schizophrenia and Personality Disorder can be at fitting a stereotype. It's easy for people to see the stereotype and not, each patient as a unique individual.

Whole Life

Michaela makes a point that most of us are fortunate enough to have a balanced lifestyle: we split our time between family, work and friends and look after not only our physical wellbeing but also our mental wellbeing in a wider community. She very reasonably asked why is it when we work with those with mental health problems we tend to focus on symptoms and treatment alone. After treating the person, we see their mental health improve and have attempted to send them on their way, sometimes back into the same situation that led to their problems in the first place. Her argument — Whole Life isn't rocket science, its plain old common sense — is a valid one. It's about being aware of all aspects of a person's life, not just their signs and symptoms. She says for many years and with good intentions, mental health workers tried to provide activities, friendships and clubs for people with mental health problems but by doing this within the 'asylum' segregation is maintained. The Whole Life philosophy is articulated and infused into the philosophy of Bowman and attempts to redress these issues. The team have worked hard to develop partnerships with Cornwall College, and with housing and leisure providers in order to provide activities using local services and facilities the public access.

Continuity of care

In order to understand what happens with our men, it was interesting to again reflect on my own experience. I was about to head back to New Zealand for Christmas on a 20 - 30 hour long haul flight. Having done a lot of driving recently, I was aware of my niggling lower back. I knew I should return to Liz, my chiropractor but I was embarrassed as she had suggested a list of exercises which I didn't do. I knew I should have and I knew they would have helped. When I was seeing her regularly, it was easy. Her treatment helped. Somehow, even though I knew this would happen, I let maintenance and my exercises slip and my pain returned. Regular contact with the same person (even if they are paid to do a job) helps. You do all sorts of things you wouldn't imagine you might do, or could do. When you think you are well, you stop treatment and the problem recurs. My back is fine and I'm heading back to the chiropractor just before I leave on yet another long haul flight. I am learning the therapeutic relationship is often the tool for enabling health.

Changing named nurses

Here is a seemingly straight forward issue that raised some discussion and a potential split in the team.

One of the men made a request to change his named nurse. I was not prepared to consider this while he was behaving aggressively. Some members of the team felt he would be getting his own way again. Aware of the split, it was important to listen for the quiet comment and typically it was made by one of the quieter staff members. We were reminded we wouldn't have the same difficulty if this person had schizophrenia rather than a personality disorder. Once we recognised this, there was an improvement and we were able to consider a change. The person began to have a more reasonable adult relationship with Carol and she was able to discuss the matter with him. However he still wanted a change of named nurse. As a team we wanted to let him know we were considering this. We also knew it would effect the other men who had formed working relationships and they would also need to change their named nurse. In the end, he decided to stay with the 'devil he knows'.

He had been listened to and thought about and that was the difference.

Weight

Weight is an issue for our men. Not all of them, but when it was present, it was often strikingly so. I had somewhat crassly approached this by putting together what I called 'A Fat Pack' and 'A Fit Pack'. To the men's credit they treated it as they should have, with hurt and disinterest. I think we are a little bit better at managing this but I'm not quite sure what we have done. Through the community meetings, we have talked about weight and health and when the request was made for increasing the number of takeaway nights from one to two. It included the provision that if men were putting on weight, this would return to one night a week only. It was the men themselves who pointed out blanket rules for everyone was unfair, and as with other parts of our practice, it needed to be individualised. Interestingly the men accepted this, and didn't become involved in competitive rivalry. Catch also made it clear we should be definite about there being two slices each and not two loaves of bread available with the evening meal, there weren't second helpings, and if a takeaway was being had that night, then the evening meal wasn't available as well. It is hard with a chronic population who seem to have so little, and it is tempting to acquiesce to requests for the simple pleasures in life. As a whole I think we manage this reasonably well. Alongside this we have an outdoor orientated focus to increase exercise and we hope to recruit and appoint a person for this in the near future.

Got a Light?

Smoking. Virtually everywhere I have worked cigarettes, tobacco, lighters and having enough money to purchase these is part of psychiatric unit life. Although there are now designated smoking areas, the requests haven't changed. Various quit programmes are offered with the usual augmentation aids but with little commitment.

I'm not a smoker, but am aware of nicotine's addictive properties, as I experienced my wife giving up the habit! I am a doctor but I also had to accept Marg was an adult able to make her own choices. Quite hard when it's someone you love and know is going to become unwell. Marg has now been on Nicorette for 15 years, hasn't smoked and hasn't had pneumonia again. It's been worth it.

Recently Carol and Siva have developed a physical health clinic. As part of this, our men have had the opportunity to work through their own individual booklets on the cost of smoking in their lives. A few have been genuinely surprised at how much they might spend over a lifetime and what else they might have done with the money. Some have stopped. Some have cut down. Some have continued. It's not dissimilar for drugs and alcohol. Tricky isn't it?

Medical illness

The other aspect of medical care is the indirect effect of attending to medical morbidity.

It wasn't until I started to attend to Tom's liver status which I had somehow put on the back burner, that he began to engage with the service. He appeared genuinely grateful I would take the time to take a history, examine him, take blood tests and refer him to a consultant hepatologist for review. I think this enabled him to begin to settle on the unit, and not be so insistent on leaving or absconding when he was on leave. He was beginning to get the sense we were genuinely interested in his care. It is perhaps the same phenomena I have noticed when engaging with families. It was not because it was on a checklist for 'best practice', but because there was a genuine interest in wanting to meet this person's family. There was an appreciation on the men's part that we seemed to accept their family, rather than judge, criticise, lament or change them.

The real world

And finally, our social inclusion officer's account of a recent incident in the community, highlights our men have feelings too.

Acceptance

One of the men on the unit, Mark went to a local shop to buy something. While in the queue he totally misunderstood the shop assistant as she did him. He threw a pork pie back on to the counter which bounced off hitting the store manager in the back. Words were exchanged, Mark stormed out. As a result was banned from the shop! On his return to the unit he was really angry about this and was adamant it was all her fault, that she had really cheesed him off and he wasn't sorry about it!

I wondered which shop assistant had been involved. I had met one of them and she was often preoccupied or just plain rude. Before I approached Mark to get to the bottom of the incident and to ask him to apologise, I asked one of the other men what he thought about that particular shop assistant. His reaction was, "She's an old bag and asked me to show my money before I bought something." Hmm, interesting.

I went to Mark and asked him if he could tell me his side of the story. He said while he was in the queue she pulled a face at him, mumbled something to the lady in front who moved and tried to hide the cash machine from him. I told Mark even if she was rude, he couldn't throw the pie at her. If you don't care because you think you're only some crazy fool from the hospital, what chance does anyone have? After talking about how he felt and what we needed to do, Mark was able to say how he was hurt. He decided to offer to pay for the pork pie but wouldn't come with me to talk it through with them.

I went to see the shop manager to get their point of view. I told him it appeared to me it was clearly a misunderstanding on both sides. I felt it was as much their fault as Mark's inappropriate behaviour. As Mark doesn't have a bank card he doesn't know about 'chip and pin' and even though he shouldn't have reacted in that way, nor should the assistant because he's from the hospital. It really doesn't mean anything other than he has a mental health problem. He is very self aware and she clearly made him feel worthless, upset and very hurt by the whole incident.

I gave them Mark's money for the pie and insisted they take it although they were reluctant. As a lesson to Mark he didn't even get the pie to eat. They agreed to lift his ban and let him into the shop again. Once back on the unit I told Mark it was up to him if he went back there. He spent the rest of the afternoon in tears and was very upset by the whole incident. In his head he felt it showed how he's not accepted. Consequently he felt really bad about himself. I was pleased I had taken that one step further and hoped the shop assistant recognised her unfair actions were a large part of the problem.

A few days later I went to the shop. The manager

told me Mark had been in and had told them he was glad they had reconsidered banning him, but if it was to happen again he would take his business elsewhere. I couldn't help but laugh, but in effect Mark retrieved some dignity and self worth.

I read this section to Mark to make sure he was happy with what was being said about him and the incident. He said later, he knew it was wrong as he had misread the actions and regretted losing control and had apologised. This incident highlights the difficulties and sadness our men and their families experience in the community.

So what of our men? As discussed elsewhere, Paul over a six month period, gradually progressed to Fettle House rehabilitation unit, despite some initial anxieties and hesitancies. Zach managed to progress directly to a supported accommodation. It was interesting to see the importance to him, of being able to return to our unit for daily medication over a period of several months. His attachment to our secure base was significant. Similarly with Mr A who had survived a relapse in the community. He had returned to our unit and was discharged again with a more robust community package in place. It was his ongoing and spontaneously initiated phone calls to let us know he had arrived safely, he had taken his medication, or the train was delayed and he was running late, that indicated this attachment.

In contrast to standardised one size fits all models of care which would be presumably well intentioned, the focus nowadays is very much on individual preferences - 'whatever it takes'. Sarah, our social inclusion officer, spent time discussing a project with input from the elder care wards on how to put together a person's life story. We wanted to do the same, inviting each of the men to contact their family, introduce us to their families, get photos of them when they were younger, and as they grew up, and went to school – ie when they were people and not patients. The men had an opportunity to choose their own duvet covers to personalise their rooms. Lee had a lovely photo of himself holding his baby nephew that stood in pride of place in his bedroom. Tony had his steam train books and models in his room as this was an important part of who he was as a person.

Others weren't so fortunate. Mark (the name he chose by this man who didn't want to use his own name) had been in various forms of institutional care from the age of seven onwards. At times it was quite difficult to connect with him and I sought advice from one of my colleagues. She suggested maybe I had inadvertently hurt, offended or had not been there for him in some way. His trust in others was likely to be critical and it was important he had control of how close anybody could ever get to him. I went up and apologised to him. I would like to be able to tell you this made a difference, but I'm not sure. Over the continuing months he would occasionally appear pleasant towards myself and the other staff, thanking them for taking him into town or being delighted that when he went into town, he could buy sausages and chips instead of fish and chips. He made a trip to Asda and bought some new clothes which he seemed pleased with, but largely kept himself to himself. It must be quite an isolated existence. As staff, we are able to talk, laugh, joke, discuss, share and explore different ideas and different struggles we have, both within and outside the workplace. This doesn't seem to happen for our men. Instead they seemed to attach themselves to the staff rather than to each other. It seems sad that Mark, although making use of some of the individualised care available, was likely to remain set in his patterns and would ultimately settle in a long-term, residential care facility. As a postscript - something changed. When I talked to him about the book and asked if he was okay about signing a consent form, he was delighted. When I asked him to write the name he would like me to use he changed it and wrote his own name, Vince. When I asked him whether he would like me to read to him the parts where he was mentioned, he smiled and said "I trust you." I was touched.

Hope from Siva, our rotation registrar.

Siva

Audacity, intrepid, bold and unwilling to bow to convention. These are the sentiments I feel when thinking about my experience with Bowman Unit. The desire to be brave and the temerity to be

240

optimistic and even hopeful. To be different, to try perhaps unconventional methods requires a different mindset but most importantly it requires audacity.

Prior to my Bowman days, my view of low secure services was quite different. Here I imagined austere buildings reminiscent of the asylum days, where patients were kept locked away from the public due to their mental illness and the danger they posed to people at large. It was a place where I thought, medication was the main weapon in the battlefield and casualties were to be expected. Individuality would have no place. Structure, regime and order would rule. Hope seemed but a flickering candle on its last bit of wick. Not so with Bowman.

Some say one person can make a difference. With this unit, it's ONE TEAM can make a difference. From the moment you walk into the building you get the impression of a home rather than a hospital. Individual rooms with televisions and even games consoles. Music playing. Paintings adorn the walls. Laughter and cheeky good humour seem to be the norm rather than the exception. Here is a place where individuality is celebrated and used as a tool. Here is a place where recovery isn't just a buzz word and medication is not necessarily the only solution. It is a place that engenders hope, kindness and the feeling of being part of a family.

Here is the place where I learnt guidelines and medication, although useful are just one part of the solution. I learnt the importance of hope, the willingness to try new non-pharmacological approaches and to appreciate every patient has a story waiting to be told and in that story lies the key to recovery. The only thing required was the bravery and audacity to try something different. That is probably the most important thing I learnt and will not soon forget. It is Bowman's gift to me.

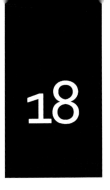

18 Maintaining compassion

Here's an account from Jess followed by Paul's own account.

Jess

We experienced a very serious incident on the unit in which a member of staff was assaulted. We are an incredibly close team and were really shocked and upset something so serious had happened to one of our colleagues who we hold in great affection. One may assume working in these environments we expect and are prepared for serious incidents. In many ways we are, but when it actually happens it's still very shocking.

It happened during a night shift and I was on shift the following day. The aftermath was surreal. Absolute shock and disbelief of what had happened and great concern for our colleague who at that time we had only heard was at a general hospital. I experienced a whole range of emotions, I felt concerned for Paul and I was relieved he hadn't been seriously injured and also selfishly relieved it hadn't been me.

I felt scared it had happened without any obvious trigger or warning signs. I felt concern, disappointment and sadness for the man who had assaulted Paul and guilty for not resenting him for what he had done and confusion as to why I felt this way.

Then, there was the concern for what would happen to the patient who had carried out the attack. He had strongly fixed delusional beliefs that he was regularly being attacked by others in his bedroom at night. Many felt he rarely had a moment when he did not have these experiences. He was also bright, jovial and affectionate and few couldn't help feeling affection for him. There was no argument from anyone that this assault demonstrated he needed additional security and containment. It felt strange coming on shift and nursing someone in seclusion who I felt exactly the same as usual towards yet knowing what he'd done just hours before. It wasn't as if he was highly disturbed. Rather he was calm, as if he had not done anything unusual. In his mind it was justified for his own protection and yet one of our colleagues was really hurt as a result. It was difficult to identify how I felt. I felt sad and did not like the idea of him being secluded and moved out of county, but knew it was best for him.

Paul

On the evening of Friday, 7 November 2008 while supervising a medication round with a student nurse, I was stabbed in the head with a biro pen by one of the patients in an unprovoked attack.

In writing this I am aware I have become self-conscious about the dramatic nature of the sentence but without going into exact detail, this is what happened. When I think about the incident now, a year and a half later, I am struck by my immediate actions once I realised what had happened and how strange they seem now, even to me.

At the time I was calm and able to direct the team I was working with that night as to what I wanted to happen, both in terms of securing a safe unit and dealing with my own injury which looked worse than it eventually turned out to be. When I eventually left the unit and was driven to Treliske Hospital's A&E department I remember saying I would be back two nights later. The realisation of what had happened did not sink in as quickly as you might expect. In fact this turned out to be months later rather than days or weeks. Funny things stay in my mind about the night like attempting to get out of the hospital into the car park. The doors were all locked and we had to go all the way through the hospital and up through the car park to find the car. Then the rush down the A30 to Truro and eventually Treliske Hospital, then spending about three to four hours watching repeats of Star Trek – The Next Generation in the A&E waiting room all the while holding a blood soaked cloth to my head... I bloody hate Star Trek. Watching other people come in and get seen before me was odd because there I was with what looked to me a worse injury than others seemed to have and a head injury to boot... just goes to show appearances can be deceptive.

It was a relief when the duty doctor told me I only had one wound because I had been convinced the assault was of a frenzied nature. The brief glimpse I got of it even before I knew what had happened was of the patient standing over me making 'stabbing' motions, I didn't feel or see anything in his hands. The student saw him drop what turned out to be the pen and he turned and walked back to his room laughing. It was at this point I thought of his risk history and put my hand to my head. My palm was red when I looked at it and I said to my colleague "bloody hell, he's stabbed me." The next moment really felt like a movie as warm blood ran down my head.

The student was a star that night, keeping me company all the way through and eventually taking me home in the early hours. I don't think it occurred to me on the night how it had affected her but, speaking to her in the days and weeks that followed I began to understand how frightening it had been to witness the incident. To this day it is something that bonds us. It's not every day you have to tell your wife you've been stabbed at work.

The next two weeks I was off work. These were strange, most of the time I felt okay. All the staff were phoning me up and asking if I was okay and if they could do anything for me. I was the centre of attention for awhile and the talk of the hospital... apparently!!

At times however, during this period I felt low, especially the day after going to the police station with Michaela to give a statement and have photographs taken of my head. This trip to the police station turned out to be a three hour affair and I was really glad Michaela had come with me because I don't think I could have answered all the questions. The next day I felt drained, when my car wouldn't start, I went back inside, went back to bed and stayed there for the day. Also during this period, I had times where I questioned myself, did I do anything to provoke it, say the wrong thing maybe and although I was re-assured by everyone that it was a totally unprovoked attack these thoughts continued going through my head for some time.

Strangely I felt no anger to the patient, he was

very ill, probably more so than any of us thought at the time and I liked him. He was transferred to another hospital and that night was the last time I saw him. Shame really as he'd made good progress and was having unescorted leave with his family for the first time in about nine years or something. Being his named nurse as well was an extra bonus, in that I felt I was contributing in a positive way to his recovery.

One of the main things which struck me at the time was that I didn't feel a thing. I had obviously heard and read in the papers, stories about people being stabbed and not actually knowing they had been for a minute or two but had always thought they must have been exaggerating a bit to dramatise the story, but it was true. A biro isn't even that sharp is it?

Some months later in 2009 I had probably my lowest thoughts about the incident... all of my thoughts at the time returned but though I recognised how lucky I was, thoughts of what could have happened if the pen had been angled slightly different or been an inch or so lower into my temple area. As it was, the pen had gone in down the side of my head lacerating but not penetrating the skull which I suppose was sheer luck at the end of the day. I know I was lucky really because it could have been a lot lot worse.

Any nurse who has suffered an attack at the

hands of a patient they are looking after will tell you it is quite a private thing which only they have to live with. I have never been one of those nurses who thinks we will not be abused or assaulted by those we are caring for, especially on a psychiatric unit where the whole range of human emotions are often escalated to extreme levels. This incident wasn't the first and probably won't be the last I have been involved in but it is the people around you who pull you through, pick you up, and encourage you to carry on. Mental health people have a dark sense of humour, it helps us cope with the things we see and deal with on a daily basis, it definitely worked for me. Working on Bowman I knew I was lucky enough to have the best team around me.

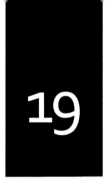

19 Saying Goodbye

There were cards, a cake. Sometimes the men would choose a barbecue on the unit or at the beach when it was time for them to leave. There were mixed feelings - for some it was clear there was the possibility of a brighter future with less restrictions and opportunities to continue becoming involved in the community. For others this would not be the case. The relationships they had formed and the safe, home-like environment where they had spent the last few years was going to be replaced by a less 'recovery and rehabilitation' focused residential setting. The men knew it. We knew it. It was sad and only briefly mitigated by our outreach capability, follow-up Christmas cards after they had left and the inevitable finite resources of the community teams.

Tips for discharge from hospital

I'm not quite sure where we got these; I think it may have been when I was in Tasmania. Anyway it seemed good, sound, practical, sensible advice and we try and remember to give it to our men when they leave. I have also added some tips for surviving homelessness from The Big Issue. Again I like it as it came from a different experience base than my own and therefore had a genuineness and practicality about it.

251

"Discharge from hospital is a time when we all react differently. Some feel very happy, others may be scared they will be unable to cope when they leave, and some have mixed feelings. It is a change and therefore a stress, so here are a few points to help you to help yourself. Some points may be irrelevant to you, so take what you feel you need and leave the rest. Everyone is unique so some of these tips may or may not be useful, but it might help to encourage those who read this to devise their own way of dealing with discharge.

- Don't expect to be cured totally when you go home. You may not be fully recovered and need support by a community team. We are not exempt from life's joy and sorrows or from the outside environment, so put you first, and practice stress management and patience. You are the most important person in the world to you.

- If you don't have a doctor, ask your mental health service to help you find one with whom you feel you connect and trust.

- Please don't stop taking your medication for any reason (possibly you don't feel you need it any more or you hate the side effects etc). PLEASE take what the doctor has prescribed for you and if you are unhappy about the medication, talk to your doctor. If you stop taking it when you go home or even reduce it on your own, it may cause you more suffering and hospitalisation in the future.

- Pace yourself. Take care of yourself. If something

needs to be done urgently, take small steps to complete it.

- Realise it takes a while to get sick so it will take a while to feel better. If you do this then you don't need to put great expectations on yourself or put yourself down or lose hope – because there is hope.

- People like family or friends may not listen to you or talk with you in the same way as in hospital. If this is hard for you, try to accept we cannot change other people and there are professionals in the community you can talk to just like the ones who have taken care of you while you were in hospital.

- Try not to start changing your whole life at once (even feeling 100% on the day of returning home) eg accommodation, jobs, voluntary work etc as it will increase your stress level. In other words, take it EASY until you feel strong enough to gradually change what you need to. Prioritise.

- If you have been following a time of day in hospital to get out of bed, try to get out of bed immediately when you wake up at that time, because it gives you a routine. Lying in bed thinking thoughts may increase your levels of depression and decrease your motivation.

- Prejudice – someone may have misunderstood you and disappeared from your life. That is their loss. There will always be people like this so concentrate on yourself and pace yourself before you set out to make a new friend.

- Treat yourself kindly because you are precious and you have been through so much pain. If you need to lie around for a couple of days to get stronger, try not to put yourself down by thinking you are lazy.

- If you are scared of shopping because the real world may be overwhelming, take someone with you the first time you go. If this is not possible, try to concentrate on what you are buying ie concentrate on the labels, make an effort to choose different products and different prices. Concentrating on what you are doing will make it easier to ignore the other shoppers or feel overwhelmed.

- Try not to think 'if only' I could be well off or 'why has this happened to me' or 'what did I do to deserve this'. It is okay to have a whinge about an illness, but it can hold us back. The more we learn about and accept ourselves the way we are now, the more we will become comfortable in our own skin.

- Restlessness – the amount varies from person to person. If it is too much for you, even if the doctor has prescribed side effect medication, try sitting still for five minutes now and again during the day. Finding something to occupy your mind and to concentrate on for a few minutes or hours can be helpful. For example, ringing a friend, playing a computer game, watching TV, listening to a song, singing, playing a musical instrument, reading a few lines from a magazine or a book or (although we are not children) just start reading a comic. Going for a drive or taking a walk around the block can be helpful. Look at different houses, gardens, flowers and trees. Some people find craft work or outside activities helpful, so see if there is something you can enjoy.

- There is always stress involved with any changes in anyone's life and therefore you may find leaving hospital stressful. Listen to your gut feelings. If you feel uncomfortable about socialising etc, leave it until you build up your own inner strength, or make small steps like using the telephone to socialise.

- There are great positives in leaving hospital so enjoy the feeling when you get home of not being told when to eat, sleep, watch TV etc. You have been through a lot while in hospital so be kind to yourself and enjoy your new found freedom."

Nine tips for surviving homelessness

1. A good source of hot food is essential if you are homeless. Even if you had the money your health would suffer if you ate takeaway all the time, so get to know where the local soup kitchen is and where day centres are that provide a hot meal – some charge a nominal amount for meals (50p is not unusual), so don't go expecting it all for free.

2. Nobody likes a bad case of BO. Keeping clean can be a problem for homeless people. Here again is where the day centres can often help – many have a washing machine and tumble dryer as well as showers you can use, and it can feel really good to

have a nice, hot shower and clean clothes. If your local day centre isn't outfitted with washing and shower facilities, have a word with a truck driver and find out where the local overnight lorry park is, as they often have a shower and laundry block on site. It won't be free but you won't be smelly.

3. Keeping warm at night will be your biggest battle, and no matter where you crash a sleeping bag and/or blanket will be of benefit to you. If you haven't already got one go to the Salvation Army and ask them where they are distributed locally. You will probably be told they are given out by the soup runs – or they might just tell you to wait while they go and fetch you one. While you are there it might be a good idea to enquire if there are any Salvation Army run hostels in the area, as of all the hostels I've stayed in the Sally Ann was by far the best.

4. It's not just the smell of your feet that should concern you, but their condition. It's all too easy to neglect your feet. This can cause you real problems, everything from blisters and athlete's foot to trench foot or worse. If you can scrape the money together, invest in a good pair of boots such as Doc Martins. If you can't scrape much together for a new pair go and have a look around the local army surplus for a pair of second hand boots, your feet will be glad you did.

5. You will be carrying everything you own, so a good backpack is a must. These are next to impossible to lay your hands on second hand, so keep your eye

on the camping shops for a sale – with luck you should pick up an 80 litre pack for around £20 to £40.

6. No Fixed Abode? Go away. If you haven't an address to send mail to, benefits can be difficult to claim, and if a miracle happened and you were offered council accommodation where would they send the letter informing you of it? If you have someone you trust locally ask them if they mind having your mail sent care of their address.

7. As spring approaches the tourist industry wakes from its winter sleep. This can be good news for homeless people in several respects, a job and housing in one handy package. If you have any skills that could be used in hotels, holiday camps or camp sites it's time to start applying – but if you get a job, remember to save enough from your wages for a deposit on a flat at the end of the season.

8. Keep your eyes open, always keep a pen and paper handy. In your daily wanderings you will pass shops with adverts in the window, one of them could lead you to the flat of your dreams so it's worth taking a few seconds to give them a scan as you pass. If possible when ringing landlords have a number ready you can be contacted at, even if it's to tell you what time you need to ring them back again – landlords tend to be busy people, you will come across a lot of answer-phones in your quest for accommodation so try and plan out what you intend to say in advance.

9. Never give up. There are organisations out there such as The Big Issue, The Salvation Army, hostels and Shelter to name but a few who will try and get you off the streets. It might not happen today or even next week, but if you're prepared to do some of the work it's only a matter of time. Many of these organisations are charities, and most of the staff are volunteers who give their time freely for your benefit. Please bear this in mind in your dealings with them – it costs nothing to be polite, but it could make things happen for you a lot quicker and a lot smoother if you are.

Ian has now developed a 'Moving On' transitions group to prepare the men for that time. Remember Dan? He's now left, but returns to contribute to this group. We are also about to add a carer's session to the same programme. Annette speaks to the families prior to their son's admission and together we welcome and encourage visits.

"If we are facing the right direction, all we have to do is to keep on walking".

Ancient Buddhist Expression

SIX

Come on over, we're
just next door

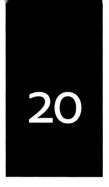

20 Belonging

We were a bit nervous about writing this chapter on families. On the one hand, we didn't want to offend or distress those families who have endured things we cannot imagine. On the other hand, we also wanted to be true to our own observations and to reflect clinical practice as we found it.

I was due to meet Tim's mum at 10.30 am. Tim, Sarah (our social inclusion officer) and I were walking over to the new podcast room just to have a look. On the way we bumped into Linda, Tim's mum. She had driven up in her little old white van. When she got out, she was different from what I expected. She was wearing a purple cap over a yellow head-band, a long black coat over a rainbow coloured dress and black Doc Martin boots. We had spoken a couple of times on the phone. She said she had previously made complaints against the service and expressed the view that Tim needed to be looked after long-term because two previous attempts at management in the community had failed. She also said she hadn't been able to visit Tim in hospital because her other son had been accidentally killed the day before Tim's admission to Bowman Unit, and described a long-standing conflict with her ex-husband.

It was strange to have our first face-to-face meeting while walking across disused hospital grounds past a plot of land with an old greenhouse on, and over to the podcast room. I still wasn't quite sure whether to ask Linda to contribute to this book but decided to take the leap anyway. Her approach and experience made me glad I did. Hopefulness, inspiration, astute observations and as it transpired, remarkable enthusiasm and connections made the risk more than worthwhile and enabled me to begin this chapter.

I think what impressed me was Linda's honesty. Yes, the families shared the observations which had been made, namely that people's backgrounds were complex and difficult, Linda suggested the phrase "dysfunctional families." She added that this phrase had also been used as part of a blaming culture. She began to describe the struggle she had experienced over the time it took to diagnose Tim and how people seemed unable to see her son as a person. Instead she would regularly go to meetings where comments were made "Tim did this or Tim didn't do that" focusing on his behaviour rather than upon positive things that happened, the value of art, the value of hope, the value of doing things differently. Tim cried. As we wandered back to the unit, Linda paused to pick up a worm on the asphalt and flicked it into the garden, making the comment she felt sorry for worms when they were stranded. Bohemian and unexpectedly remarkable. Linda sent us this for our book.

A mother's perspective – reflections on the effects of my son's mental ill health.

My son is 36 years old now. Since he was 18 he has spent many years detained in psychiatric and brain injury units, interspersed by many short-term attempts at semi-independent living, chaotic lifestyle and accompanying habits usually seeping their way back in over the course of six to 12 months, dissipating any progress made. This seemingly endless cycle of despair having a deep and lasting impact, which at times has been a test of love, understanding, endurance and loyalty.

I have witnessed and been part of many chaotic situations over the last 18 years. It is difficult to put into words the range of emotions I have experienced, difficult to imagine unless you also have a grown up child that suffers mental ill health, but try if you can to imagine witnessing somebody you love loosing themselves over and over again, my son like many other sons and daughters, being prone to lash out and attack those that love them the most... their mothers (and fathers).

It has been a long road, one that has left me weary. It has taken this length of time to accept my son will probably not ever be free in the sense I have always hoped for, I also now realise I have to take a back-seat. I cannot make him better and I need to continue to find strategies to cope with what is, I believe a never ending bereavement. I lost the son I knew because he lost himself, quite literally. One of the first labels being Schizophrenia (type 2). There have been many assessments and prognoses, made more complicated because of 'dual diagnosis' – brain injury and psychotic illness.

At last after all these years the need to attach a label seems to matter less, which I find entirely refreshing. It is important to remember my son has little insight into the causes of his condition and the consequences of his related behavioural problems. In his view, he is being endlessly punished without due cause. He is resistant and mistrustful - who could blame him?

Over these years spent 'in the system' I have seen many changes. My biggest criticism has been lack of communication between me as nearest relative/advocate/guardian and the professionals involved in his care plan. This lack of involvement adds to the feelings of helplessness, guilt and isolation. Parent's insights and knowledge of their offspring are all too often overlooked because we are not heard.

In those early years of pre-diagnosis I felt isolated, uninformed and frightened; we veered from one crisis to the next, our home life best described as armageddon. These years have had a long-term detrimental effect on my son, his younger siblings and me.

Any parent with a grown up child who has a psychotic illness will have their own story to tell, all equally harrowing and desperate. It is so important to remember it is not anyone's fault. Guilt can only add to the already too much to bear despair of watching somebody you love and want to protect go through such pain.

I realise now I have spent years responding to and perpetuating patterns of behaviour which are not based on rational thought processes but it is a mother's instinct to care for her child, especially if that child happens to be a vulnerable adult.

I am still not sure where the boundary lines are but it was once said to me by a carer's support worker that "I have a right to my own life." I have tried to keep this in mind when times get tough, which they often do, because it is true. I think all carers should try and remember this. I believe just considering it helps to preserve and strengthen the self. I have copied the following diary of events.

Sunday 6/5/01

Tim returned to the house after an all day

drinking session with his half brother. He woke his younger brother (asleep on the sofa), with a start by putting two fingers up his nose. A struggle developed which turned into a verbal dispute. I intervened and a few moments later Tim physically attacked his brother who was still lying on the sofa. This shocked his brother enough to make him break down, he didn't fight back, he was too frightened. I eventually pulled him off and Tim rushed upstairs swearing and shouting abuse. We were both in a state of shock and I felt it necessary to ring the out of hours emergency community psychaitaric nurse (CPN). During this conversation I was aware Tim was listening in on his phone upstairs.

My partner went upstairs to see and hear Tim shouting abuse at the nurse. He was extremely angry and when it was suggested he shouldn't speak to anybody in that manner he threw the phone across the room. He also threw his mobile phone across the room and started to lash out, hitting the door with his fist with such force he broke a bone in his hand. Just previous to this he had kicked a kitchen unit door in. Tim eventually admitted he hadn't been taking his medication; he agreed to take it along with some painkillers for his hand. Tim was still very anxious that the police would be coming and was shouting out what he would do to them if they came. A doctor arrived (with three policemen who stayed downstairs) and examined his hand. It was decided the situation was not serious enough to admit him for assessment (which I disagreed with).

The next day, Bank Holiday Monday he was still edgy, threatening to kill his sister's kitten and have his sister evicted. On the Tuesday, after having his hand seen to at hospital he was advised by the doctor, during an emergency appointment, that he should go into hospital to be reassessed. He was transferred to the unit as a voluntary patient.

Saturday 12/5/01

I rang the unit at about 8.30 pm to have a word with Tim and to see how he was; he was with the doctor so I spoke to a nurse. She said he had been stressed with the noise in hospital and he thought he would be better off at home. He was granted leave till Tuesday and was going to get the 9.00 pm train back to home. I queried the fact that this would mean Tim would be alone in the house on Monday with his younger brother because I work on that day. As Tim had physically attacked him the previous Sunday, I didn't feel it was safe for Tim to be alone with him. It was agreed Tim would go back to the unit on Monday.

Tim arrived back home having been given a lift by a nurse from the unit. We all sat down and talked for a while. Tim appeared to be restless, and agitated raising and lowering the sunglasses, which he had previously swapped for his stereo system (worth £200) from his half brother who had visited him that afternoon. The nurse left and almost as soon as he departed Tim became abusive, put a record on at high volume and started to rant and swear initially at me. I asked him if when he had gone out they had had a drink. This question provoked an extreme reaction, which began to be directed at my other son, my partner and especially at myself.

His objection was that he didn't want to be questioned by his mother about whether he had had a drink that afternoon. This developed into a full-scale verbal attack directed at all of us. The essence of his objections was that he didn't want to live in the same house as us, that it was restricting living here.

His behaviour was threatening, his language vile and abusive. Our response was to attempt to calm the situation by talking to him but this didn't work so we tried to remove ourselves from his presence by going into other rooms several times. He wanted all three of us to get out of 'his' house (he has a 45% stake in the house as a result of the compensation from his accident). Despite asking us to leave and demanding to be left alone he followed us from room to room shouting abuse. He seemed to believe there was a conspiracy against him, to have him sectioned. I told him I would ring the unit and speak to a nurse. He didn't want me to but I felt I had to because the situation was threatening and out of control, on the verge of physical violence. He had been back home less than an hour.

When the police arrived his anger was directed at them, they agreed to take him in to the unit despite having a car rather than a van. They requested he was accompanied for safety reasons. He reluctantly agreed to be taken in after kicking the car and shouting abuse. During the journey he spat on the floor of the car and continued to be abusive to the police who showed considerable restraint.

When Tim received his compensation in February 2000, we decided it was worth pooling resources and buying a house where Tim could be semi-independent in rooms of his own. The alternative was for Tim to buy a house and live by himself; this was felt by all parties to be unrealistic. Previous to this, the years Tim had spent in safe houses usually resulted in him spending half the week in the family home because he wasn't happy. The decision to live in the same house seemed to be the best solution.

It's apparent this situation has not worked and that another way forward needs to be found. We have tried very hard to make Tim happy but

I acknowledge now we have failed and that we are in a destructive situation that cannot go on, I have to think about the rest of my family. The situation is desperate enough for me to consider selling the house (in order to pay Tim back his share) and to relinquish responsibility as Tim's receiver.

Thurs 17/5/01

I returned from shopping at 5.45 pm to find Tim's rucksack in the front-room. I went up to his attic and found him lying on his bed. I asked him why he had come home and he wouldn't answer. I went downstairs to listen to a message from the unit asking if I would ring them, which I did. I was told he had barged out of the unit as two people were entering without waiting for the doctor to arrive to make an assessment.

Tim came down as I was on the phone and started laying the law down telling me to get out of his house, his brother was still asleep in his room so when I saw my daughter off to work (I reassured her it was ok for her to still go to work despite her concern). I rang my sister using a mobile phone from outside the house as we were on our own. My sister arrived quite quickly to find Tim verbally threatening me. We both tried to reason with him without success and he became aggressive and frightening. We felt the best thing to do was to get out the house quickly for our own safety. We drove a short distance up the road so he thought we had gone and rang the police. My partner arrived shortly before the police and after a short discussion we all went to the front door, which had been locked. Strangely Tim opened the door and we all went in. The police along with my partner, tried to reason with Tim for about 10-15 minutes but the discussion was going no-where. When one of the police officers took him by the arm (not the one with plaster-cast) he started to lash out. There was a struggle and he was restrained. In the struggle the sofa he was sitting on went backwards slightly and touched a large pane of glass, which shattered. Luckily the venetian blind was down and this prevented glass coming into the room. However a small piece of glass which had landed on the sofa cut Tim slightly on the right-side of his head. Because Tim had a plaster-cast on his right hand he was turned over and a plastic restraining tie was used instead of handcuffs. During all of this Tim was swearing and shouting abuse at the police. Once again we were all left shocked and traumatised by what had happened and deeply concerned about Tim's mental state.

Linda (Tim's Mother)

The long awaited hope (Nicola)

When I first met with family members I only heard negatives. I wanted to hear something positive to hold on to; there was nothing. I became a 'workaholic' in my business just to cope and it wasn't until Debbie was able to ask "What are you doing to yourself?" I realised what I'd done.

I had spent many years visiting my son in various different secure hospitals which were dotted throughout the UK. Each new location would be interspersed with brief periods of hope when he would be discharged, only for his mental health to quickly deteriorate again, followed by yet another round of reviews and then – finally – the inevitable upset of another section order.

First Exeter, then Reading followed by Manchester, then back to Cornwall and finally back again to Exeter – it seemed no matter what care was offered, some other hospital was always necessary for Dean's next step. When I was informed Bowman would be opening in Bodmin – a mere 30 miles away – I was elated. We were almost counting down the days after his initial assessment and being told Dean had been accepted.

I had a meeting with Michaela (the unit manager)

and attended the open-day a few weeks later. I was unexpectedly nervous and dreaded the thought of having to go through the routine of getting to know yet another team of staff. I was greeted at the doors by Catch – who to my relief, I already knew from a couple of years ago when Dean had been a patient on the neighbouring Harvest Unit.

My first impression of most of the staff I met was of a warm and friendly group of professionals – and I was particularly struck by a new social worker who sadly left after just a few months. This happens a lot and I always find it difficult when the person who leaves is someone who has a positive influence on your child's care. She assisted Catch in showing me around the unit and demonstrated the facilities that were already in place, telling me what else they were hoping to have installed on the unit in the future.

I have to admit my first impression of Bowman Unit itself was very mixed. It was a lovely, light unit with wide passageways and good rooms for the patients – but I couldn't believe how small the unit felt and I was struck by the widely mixed age group and the different degrees of illness the patients on the unit exhibited. What would these men do with their time in such close proximity to each other? Especially at that time, as there was not even a pool table or other social distractions for them.

However I pushed any negative thoughts to the back of my mind and thought "Let's just see what happens!" Our main priority was to have Dean back in Cornwall and close to his family. It meant such a huge difference to him knowing we were only 45 minutes from Bowman, instead of being hundreds of miles and hours and hours of driving away.

I soon built up a very good rapport with the staff involved in Dean's care and I think they quickly came to realise he came from a very closely knit family. I found it was easy to establish a good clear line of communication with staff like Iain and Catch, both of whom were directly involved in Dean's care and this made my situation more at ease. They gave me clear and regular updates of an ever changing situation – something that is vital as my son's illness can exhibit so differently and on an almost daily basis.

Over the last two years it's turned out the staff and Dean have really begun to gel. This is something I haven't seen with Dean over the last eight years of hospitalisation and I started to wonder what it was that is so different in this unit. Over the years I have spent time with various different members of staff, in various different units and in wildly differing scenarios, but I've never seen Dean so comfortable in his carer's presence.

I have to admit I am aware the staff must have initially thought of me as an ogre! I love my son very deeply and will do anything to ensure he is well cared for and as happy as it is possible for him to be. It gradually became apparent though that Dean was finally treated as a normal human being and not just as a patient or a daily chore to be tolerated.

Dean's struggle and constant battle with his thought disordered illness is ongoing with no let-up and we all were very aware this was going to be a challenge and a half. Over time we gradually saw this dark cloud of bizarre thoughts and emotions that surround Dean starting to lift. We saw him beginning to laugh and smile and be himself – slowly turning back into the son I had lost so many years ago.

This is something I have hung onto to this day. I really believe Dean's improvement is due to the constant support and never-give-up attitude that flows from the team on Bowman Unit. We, as Dean's family, often have a laugh and keep reminding ourselves no one is perfect in the world and there is no real definition of 'being normal'. Everyone has a certain special gift to give and Dean's is his warmth towards his family.

We don't want to be disparaging or judgemental of families who have had the experiences they have had.

There does appear to be something characteristic about the families and it is difficult to know how best to describe this. We meet with as many families as we can, in part to introduce ourselves as the people looking after their son, and in part to get to know more about the men as people with their own stories. We felt it might be important for the men to know their families were important to us. Our sense is that somehow this has been appreciated. That we took an interest in their families and therefore saw them as individuals somehow contributed to their engagement, to the shift from the 'us and them' culture and of being genuinely interested in the person while remaining aware of their illness and index offence.

So what were the similarities? These families had both had more than their fair share of difficulties. How do you continue to visit and love your son who, when unwell, had done something awful? How do you manage at Christmas time when your own mother has said the only contact she wishes to have is if her son should die? What must have happened to lead to that state of affairs?

How do you manage as a single mother when your son is falling behind at school, using illicit substances, becomes violent and then develops not only schizophrenia but a treatment resistant schizophrenia? How does the young man learn when their father has been absent and their mum hasn't been able to say and mean "No"? How does he manage when he comes onto a unit where there aren't so many mixed messages? Then when he goes home for a visit, Mum keeps saying it's fine when it isn't. Even though we try to support mum to be able to tell us what is really happening, she feels unable to do so. After having the discussion, we too are left, as the young man is, not knowing what mum really means when she says "It's okay."

What if the man who, through his mother's own schizophrenia, was taken into care at the age of seven? We had difficulty knowing what he was thinking and feeling. What must it have been like for a seven year old trying to understand and relate to his own mother? Other mums were able to say they had been "gullible". They had believed what their sons had said and had tried to protect them from the things that might hurt them but things may have also stopped them from learning from life. It's complicated. As parents we get up in the morning and try to do our best.

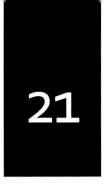

21 Tribunals and other legal matters

What a nightmare! I sat in two tribunals the other day, (one of them may have been a manager's review), where over 50 hours of combined professional time had been tied up and paid for without a single benefit for either patient. A colleague suggested to me that these forums allow the person an opportunity to have their views heard and that this is an important part of the process. Hmm. Perhaps, but it's curious. Having worked in two other Commonwealth Countries, this neither occurs nor does there appear to be any obvious difference for the men or of abuses of the Mental Health Act. To their credit, some of our men seem to recognise this inherent wastefulness and don't attend.

I was particularly concerned when I worked here five years ago. We did write something about it and if nothing else, writing enabled me to be aware of my role, namely to provide what I hoped was an opinion. Ultimately however it was for the panel to decide. It was with refreshed interest I read a chapter on the legal process as it applies to mental health. It is so well written, I want to quote it at some length. It enabled me to settle more readily into the role and hopefully is written in such a way that the interested reader may pursue the remainder of the text for themselves. She starts off with this lovely introduction:

"It is common knowledge among criminal lawyers that most defendants would, if they could, prefer to be represented by Horace Rumpole, not only because the tense courtroom drama (including of course a sharp healthy contempt for the trial judge) is followed by the assured acquittal, but because (usually) en route Rumpole dismembers limb by limb, the testimony of the pompous expert witness. His ability to expose the professional for public humiliation is unsurpassed. While criminal lawyers may not go so far as to admit to wanting to be Rumpole, most would confess to wanting his legendary forensic skill." Lovely isn't it!

She continues, "The purpose of cross examination is to cast doubt on an expert's opinion. The manner in which this is done if at all, will depend on the skill of the advocate. The approach may be by way of a wolf in sheep's clothing that elicits extra, useful facts that put on question the factual material on which the opinion is based. This is often followed by questions designed to maximise the expert's discomfort before a life line was thrown in the form of a question such as 'of course doctor, had you known about the patient's drug abuse would you have come to the same conclusion?' – that enables the expert to retract his opinion and save face.

Or the approach may resemble the slash and burn method of farming, in the course of which sight is lost of the fact it is the evidence and not the witness personally, that needs to be discredited.

If the facts in the case are not an issue, counsel will try to place a different interpretation upon them by challenging the expert's reasoning, methods and experience. Questions put to an expert will tend to be 'closed' questions requiring specific answers which enable counsel to control the direction of cross examination. Leading questions (that suggest the answer) may be asked and counsel will generally take the opportunity to state his own expert's opinion. Counsel will attempt to undermine any opinion by establishing that a particular field of expertise cannot provide a definitive answer. Hypothetical facts will often be put to an expert to test an opinion".

In her conclusion, she adds "It is not surprising that the doctor and lawyer may gaze at each other from their respective corners of the courtroom with separate degrees of suspicion. Much may be born of ignorance of the other's discipline and training. More may derive from fundamentally different approaches to the same problem. The only common ground may be the patient, for whom each wants something different".

The second author extends this argument further. She argues that although the code for crown prosecutors emphasises that crown prosecutors must be "fair, independent and objective... they must not be affected by improper or undue pressure from any source," Penelope regards these as admirable sentiments only. She suggests they are effectively "meaningless in view of the political considerations and media attention which underpin the appearance of the mentally disordered offender before the court.

In my view it is nonsensical to suggest the political profile and importance of the policy of care in the community or the baying of the press when a mentally disordered offender commits a serious offence, have no repercussions for the prosecution and the sentencing of all mentally disordered offenders". She continues saying "No judge wants to entrust the decision about when a violent mentally disordered offender is released from hospital to doctors whose primary concern is seen as one of the welfare of the patient, when it is the judge who takes the brunt of media attention if things go wrong. It is 'safer' to opt for a Section 47 Restriction Order and leave the decision to the Home Secretary. Further and complementing the public trial itself," she adds "the adversarial system is not about the search for truth. Nor is it about the unfettled disclosure to the jury of information in order to assist them in reaching the proper decision. It is about contests. It mostly involves confrontation. The trial is not designed to understand the offender or the offence, only to see whether, within the framework blame can be placed and responsibility apportioned."

She concludes "My conception of the criminal justice system is that it reflects society's attitudes to those who are mentally disordered: it views them with suspicion, fear and something little short of contempt. Alternatively it patronises them. While the political parties are competing for the 'moral high ground' as to who is 'toughest on crime', the current government is usually considering a 'three strikes and you are out' sentencing policy while insufficient beds are available to accommodate mentally disordered patients, and while prison hospital wings are so overcrowded that mentally ill prisoners are sometimes kept on ordinary wings, the future does not look good for better treatment of the mentally disordered offender. But then perhaps neither the public or the courts really want to grapple with the problems which mentally disordered offenders present. It involves after all wrestling with what can go wrong with the human mind – and therefore with what can go wrong with all of us."

Great stuff and worth retrieving and quoting at length their clearly articulated views.

However, on the other side of the coin, there are remarkable aspects to the legal process, not least of which are the people. The panel members of the tribunals and manager's reviews appear genuinely interested in the men and their progress. The law can also be surprisingly clear in its deliberations and individuals can be quite helpful to the legally inexperienced clinician. Thanks.

I tried once in a tribunal to rearrange the room whereby the patient would be at the head of the room and the panel, clinical team and the person's lawyer grouped around in a semi-circle, facing him. I had invited us to consider developing a clinical and legal framework that together would be supportive and avoid an adversarial encounter. To my surprise, no one was particularly alarmed and were happy to go along with this suggestion. Mr A said he wasn't bothered one way or the other and so we left it as it was. I might try again for it seems that although the legal profession are bound to represent their client, one of our circuit solicitors said to me he hadn't; he had represented Mr A on many occasions as he was admitted and re-admitted through the acute and psychiatric intensive care units, and knew a period of stability in a low secure unit would be in his best interests. Accordingly the solicitor didn't immediately appeal his Section 3 status as requested but waited until there had been a period of time in which he could settle into Bowman. If, we as clinicians haven't done our job by informing the tribunal as clearly and succinctly as to why the person should remain under the act, particularly when they now present as well as they do as a result of receiving compulsory treatment and containment, then their questioning ensures we attend to these details in future. To this end, one solicitor has a reputation for attending to detail. Personally I found him quite supportive and if he isn't, then very reasonably he raises differences of opinion and inconsistencies on our part. If he doesn't, then who does?

It has taken me to my last tribunal to realise maybe the panel members are frightened. Frightened that they may unnecessarily detain or frightened they will mistakenly discharge a person.

Different personalities manage this anxiety in different ways. Some wish to pay attention to the detail, exact dates, as if this may contain their fear and anxiety. Others may do so by inflaming one another in the belief that an adversarial approach will lead to truth. It's watching and understanding which member wants what and attempting to provide them with this security. Sadly the various panels seem to presume other than what is hopefully more likely, that most of us are trying to do our best in what can be difficult circumstances.

Community Treatment Orders

As we veer into a more positive note, I want to make a comment about Community Treatment Orders (CTOs). It is interesting working in different countries and seeing how each approaches various issues. We have been using CTOs in Australia and New Zealand for at least a couple of decades. Used correctly they were quite effective, particularly when the service responded decisively and the person was then able to learn they were in fact more than pieces of paper. People who had begun to deteriorate, or who had missed their depot on their due date and who had a characteristic relapse signature, could then be retrieved and their care could continue in the community. The reason I am raising the matter of CTOs is not because they are particularly contentious any longer, or at least I hope not, rather that I saw the Vendors Code of Conduct in a copy of 'The Big Issue'. I have included their fourteen items (with permission) because when I re-read them I couldn't help but compare them to my own CTOs which seem to be much more gentle and less specific and perhaps, less helpful. See what you think.

Code of Conduct

This code outlines our responsibility to you and your responsibilities to yourself, other vendors and The Big Issue. Please read through all points below, and sign to confirm that you understand them.

The Big Issue will:

- Treat all vendors with consistency and respect and provide a safe and welcoming environment;
- Help you to maximise your sales by providing a quality magazine and an effective sales strategy;
- Protect the interests of all vendors and the public by enforcing the code of conduct;
- Whenever possible, help you to access support services relevant to your needs.

I agree to:

- Only sell the current copy of The Big Issue magazine for the stated cover price.
- Accept and co-operate with staff decisions as to my

capability to sell.

- Clearly display valid Big Issue identification/uniform at all times whilst selling.
- Only sell on an authorised Big Issue pitch.
- Adhere to the Big Issue pitch system which will be sales related.
- Always supply customers with the correct change and hand-over the magazine.
- Adhere to all local by-laws whilst selling.

I agree not to:

- Obstruct the general public. This includes sitting on the pavement, being part of a gathering on the pitch or having a dog that is not under control.
- Argue or fight over pitches with other vendors or those who earn a living on the street – eg beggars, buskers, charity collectors and street traders.
- Use threatening or aggressive behaviour.
- Use offensive language, including racist, sexist or homophobic comments.
- Supply magazines to:
  - Suspended or de-badged vendors;
  - Non vendors for re-sale to the public;
  - Any vendor who appears to be under the influence of alcohol or controlled substances;
  - Any vendor who has been refused magazines from the distribution outlet.

- Beg or busk whilst wearing The Big Issue badge/uniform or holding a copy of The Big Issue magazine.
- Sell in any way associated with begging, including sitting or lying down, or using a cup or bowl to collect money.
- Sell on private property, including rail stations and trains, supermarkets, cafes, pubs, bars and restaurants.
- Sell old editions of the magazine without prior arrangement with The Big Issue.
- Sell whilst looking after children under the age of 16.
- Appear to be under the influence of alcohol or controlled substances whilst selling or buying The Big Issue.
- Sell, buy or consume illegal substances on Big Issue property or registered pitches or give advice, directions or information that will in any way help someone else to obtain them.
- Commit a crime whilst acting as a Big Issue vendor or wearing Big Issue identification or uniform.
- Behave in any manner likely to bring The Big Issue into disrepute.

I understand that:

- By breaking any of the rules in this Code of Conduct I could face temporary or permanent suspension from selling The Big Issue magazine.

- The Big Issue staff reserve the right to refuse to supply me with magazines if I break any of the rules listed above, or appear to present a risk to myself or others.
- If I stop selling for more than six months I will have to submit and sign all relevant paperwork again and undertake further training as necessary.

Signed
Date

Police on the unit

There are two other aspects of the law we wanted to write about. Police on the unit and a very clever piece of legal work on the part of our Mental Health Act team. The first matter continues in a copy of a letter we sent to our local constabulary.

Dear Sergeant

Re: Log Number xxxxx

I just wanted to write to say thank you for your recent visit to Bowman Unit.

We hope this is an exceptional rather than regular event. However we did feel it was important to send a message to the men on the unit. Specifically the two individuals who were interviewed and counselled as to the social unacceptability and undesirability of their behaviours. I understand there was one visit last year in which you also came along to interview three of our men with respect to a small amount of marijuana having been brought onto the unit.

While it is obvious our men can at times be clearly unwell and a successful prosecution is remote you may wonder whether it is worth the visit. We believe it is. It introduces the normal rules of society, reminding those individuals who might be able to be returned to live in the community there are correct ways to behave in society. It supports the staff in their work of maintaining consistency and boundaries on the unit and importantly it also removes staff from having to make judgements about whether or not to have the matter taken seriously and investigated through the appropriate channels. It is also important for families to know that clear steps are taken should it be their son who is involved.

We appreciate your men are busy and have a difficult task to do without being asked to come to a locked unit that is already staffed. However, your role, your uniform and your approach is important.

Yours

John Little, Locum Consultant Psychiatrist

Lady Justice Butler-Sloss

For the last part of this chapter we are enormously indebted to Mark and his team, Diana and Flo. What an asset having an experienced, diligent and thoughtful Mental Health Act Administration Team who just go out of their way to help. The case relates to a mother's application for obtaining discharge for her son. The case referred to is Manchester City Council v Ingram (1999) EWCA Civ 1689 and Lady Justice Butler-Sloss' judgement, being both on the money and compassionate. Shows just how the law can work.

The background to this case is that the mother was a qualified nurse with two children, her daughter who was a teacher and her son, Paul. He lived with her from birth, apart from one or two periods where for various reasons he was removed. He had also spent a period of time in a psychiatric hospital.

Mrs Ingram believed her son had suffered from mild epilepsy which was controllable by drugs and as these could be perfectly well administered by her, he should be discharged home. She was supported in the view that her son suffered from mild epilepsy by her GP and also a professor of neurology.

The opposite view was taken by Manchester City Council and their senior social worker, at least one police officer and by two consultant psychiatrists. They took the view that Paul had chronic Schizophrenia. He had a long history of hospitalisation, violence and assaults on women and because of his size and weight, he was being looked after in a secure unit for males and was nursed by males.

The judge was faced therefore with a conflict of evidence. Further the judge was clear if no order was made and Paul was discharged now or very shortly, 'he would go home to his mother, a regime of non-co-operation and refusal to give appropriate prescribed medication would result in a decline in the son's condition with the predictable result'. The judge was satisfied Paul needed treatment and concluded that 'standing back, a reasonable person, in my judgement, in Mrs Ingram's shoes, would say Paul needs psychiatrists, neurological treatment and such is necessary in the hospital environment; ...in all the circumstances, looking at it objectively, it would be wrong to deny Paul treatment' and made the order.

Lady Justice Butler-Sloss continues however: 'Mrs Ingram comes to us and says all of this is plainly wrong. She says, he is not suffering from mental illness, that the psychiatrists do not know what they are talking about and I put it like that, that this is a neurological problem and not a psychiatric problem, that psychiatrists are not trained in neurology so how can they understand what is necessary. The correct diagnosis is epilepsy, not mental illness. She says her son is quiet and reasonable. He is polite and well behaved, that there was nothing when they turned up on the 10 January to lead anyone to want to take him away and put him into hospital. This is a denial of his human rights, she says, and is a denial of his opportunity to live quietly and peacefully in the community with his mother and sister, as he has done for so many years. She points out that he went to the gym; he went to church with his sister; he was leading a semi-normal life; he needed some looking after but he was doing very well under that regime; he can read and write; he had a high IQ and the whole of what the psychiatrists are saying and the approved social worker is saying is completely untrue. She is also very concerned the judge led her to believe that at one of the hearings that he was going to let Paul out to go home and he was being critical of the way the doctor and approved social worker dealt with the case. But then on the next occasion when she did not attend, lo and behold, he changed his mind. Was he got at she says; how was it he changed his mind from what she had learnt from him on that occasion?'

Lady Justice Butler-Sloss concludes "I have to say that I do have a lot of sympathy with Mrs Ingram who has had the greatest possible difficulty in understanding that the view of the doctors and of the approved social worker is the correct view – I say the correct view because the judge heard the evidence with enormous care. He came to conclusions; he made findings a fact, and based upon the findings of fact he decided he had to allow the council to take over the duties of the nearest relative from the mother and it is perfectly obvious the mother would not do what she was asked because she cannot believe, did not then and does not now believe, that it was the right that he should be having this treatment and he ought to be at home with her.

This is a very sad case but there is no doubting at all, in my view, that this court cannot possibly interfere with it. If we did interfere with it we would aside new order, which in my view is inconceivable, that there would be a considerable number of subsequent problems, that those subsequent problems do not arise because I, for my part, think the judge was perfectly entitled to come to the conclusion to which he has come and I would dismiss this appeal."

22 Getting on with the neighbours

Just words,
Twisted and badly tempered
In the heat
Of the moment
Just angry words

Just words
Not sticks
Or sharpened stones
Piercing a broken heart
Just angry words

Sound splashes against
A sea wall of silence
And trickles down
Into a river of tears

Just words
Echoing softly sadly
And quietly
Year upon year
Only words,
Just angry words.

Ian Goral, May 1999

I'm not sure we got on with the neighbours when I was growing up. I do recall being talked about as a family and I remain wary of gossip and small mindedness. Nevertheless, I had good friends at secondary school and I still keep in contact with them, friends having always been important and very much part of an extended social network system we have continued with our family. It has brought us a lot of joy, a lot of fun and is part of our family culture. Our network now spans a large number of towns, cities and countries.

Bowman is part of a network. We don't stand alone, our neighbours are important, helping to provide a service for the men whilst they are in our care and also a care pathway afterwards. I think we would become overwhelmed and isolated if we didn't have our neighbours and while there may be ups and downs, we couldn't do our job without their support.

The very name, Bowman Unit, conjures up the possibility of an isolated, stand-alone, specialist unit. We chose to do it differently, seeing ourselves as part of a broader mental health and community system. Harvest, the psychiatric intensive care unit (PICU), is just along the corridor. I think we have had four or five referrals, men who have been shuttling back and forth between the various general adult units and psychiatric intensive care unit - their presentations complicated by treatment non-compliance, polysubstance abuse and absconding. We didn't accept one man but Nick (the consultant on the psychiatric intensive care unit) and I were able to agree to disagree on the diagnosis, and to do so professionally and amicably as colleagues, each respecting the other's viewpoint. The commissioners were in agreement and facilitated an out of county transfer. My lasting impression of the psychiatric intensive care unit, however was their willingness to help and to do so swiftly. We had become increasingly beleaguered by Peter who had been institutionalised for 30 plus years with a personality disorder. He continued to create considerable tensions on the unit, leaving staff exhausted. There was yet another incident. We went up to Harvest and asked whether they could take him until such point when he was transferred out of county. They did so immediately, without question. They supported us and I remain grateful to Marcus for his commitment to this.

The community forensic team have also played an important in their role; Andy a warm and friendly psychologist came onto the unit to work with one of our patients and continued with him after he left. Paul and Debbie, forensic community psychiatric nurses (CPNs) have known our men for many years and kept in contact with them, both through the high and medium secure services prior to their return to Cornwall. Debbie's relationship with Dean's mother was particularly important. She had found it difficult to be able to say 'no' to her son's visits, but was able to relay this message through Debbie to us.

John is an extraordinary psychologist with a willingness to provide advice and help and to do so with a genuine interest in all of those involved. His ability to think outside the box and to contribute to a policy in risk development was always warmly received, as was his willingness to come to the unit to share his experience. Mike was a very experienced forensic social worker, having worked in Cornwall for 50 years. I hope one day he will write a history of Cornwall's mental health. (Certainly talking to him reveals he has a wide range of experience and he is in a unique position to describe the changes over half a century of mental health in Cornwall). He too has a long relationship, not only with the men that he works with on our unit, but their family through various generations. Experienced, seldom rattled, he has seen a lot. Heading the community forensic team was Bernie, who too has been willing to share, provide advice and to be involved in thinking about how the service might develop. With our new psychologist starting, the shared role with Bowman and the community forensic team will add to this relationship.

Fettle House, the open rehabilitation unit just down from us, has recently been joined by Angela, a very experienced psychiatrist. She has done many things, done them well and absolutely with the patient at the forefront of her considerable charm, intellect and determination. With her help and the help of the Fettle team, men from 'the low secure unit' have had an opportunity of progressing down to Fettle, to avail themselves of their rehabilitation opportunities and to continue their progress and onward journey. Angela's "of course we have to give it a go" approach was enormously welcoming and enabled a real opportunity for a care pathway for our men to move beyond Bowman. Similarly staff from Fettle have come up to unit rounds, come up to assess our men and have developed with the men, specific activities in order to facilitate and consolidate the transition down to Fettle. They provide good feedback, letting us know how each of the men are doing in order that together we may have a united approach to support and encourage activity. I am also particularly grateful to Jan the unit secretary who has a lovely accent, and whom I always ring up to see whether or not Angela might be available for a Monday lunchtime 'hot date!'

Although it is early days, the willingness of the Cornwall drug and alcohol team (CDAT) to genuinely take an interest in our population, recognising there are some specific needs that are different from their usual population group, was also refreshing. David's willingness to develop a process by which case based learning could occur between both services was both welcomed and valued. It will be interesting to see how it progresses.

Largely through Michaela's work and subsequently taken up and continued by our social inclusion worker,

Sarah, our community neighbours include Cornwall College and The Eden Project. The willingness of both these organisations to remain involved either in the unit or to offer our men real work in their own community is 'ideal' as they say in Cornwall. Thank you.

Finally, my most important neighbour is Gill. Her engaging warm and cheeky smile welcomes us to the hospital café, as she chats with us and takes an interest. She told me recently she had been able to find a supplier for a special bread one of our men particularly liked and rang him up to let him know.

It is this sort of support, inclusion and generosity which helps.

seven

Pick a card, any card,
pick it from the top

To laugh often and much; to win the respect of intelligent people and the affection of children; to earn the appreciation of honest critics and endure the betrayal of friends. To appreciate beauty; to find the best in others; to leave the world a bit better whether by a healthy child, a garden patch or a redeemed social condition; to know that even one life has breathed easier because you have lived. This is to have succeeded.

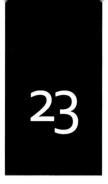

23

Do we really make a difference?

Does anything we do or have written about make any difference? It is difficult to know how to measure outcomes, but it is also important we continually attempt to do so and in so doing, refine our search for what we do that 'makes a difference'. We would like to form a consortium of low secure unit's which together could begin to explore similarities and differences between the various units. In so doing we may generate questions and with curiosity rather than competition, explore what might help. The other aspect to be aware of is of comparing apples with oranges. There is quite a nice little book, the title of which goes along the lines of "How to Lie with Statistics", the general theme being encapsulated in that title. Numbers are sneaky things. Whilst we are writing ours they need to be understood in terms of the context within which Bowman Low Secure Unit operates, socially, culturally and historically. It is with this depth and detail we are more likely to begin to unravel and understand what each unit has been able to do. The other aspect is that there are different ways of looking at outcomes and in part this is due to which set of spectacles we are wearing at the time. We have tried to present various ways of looking at outcomes rather than to focus on one to the exclusion of another. In addition to standardising measures for the unit as a whole, there is merit in individually tailoring outcome measures to a person and their specific circumstances. The acid test remains however whether we would be happy with our family member being on this unit and if not, why not? Our data isn't that clear, but for the April 2009 to March 2010, this is what we found.

A reminder

To remind you who our men are, we have attempted to collect bits and pieces of information that whilst incomplete, give you a clinical sense of who our men are and whether they might be similar or different to the men you may be working with.

The HCR-20 (which measures risk) in some ways is a convenient format for this purpose. So here goes for the men who had theirs completed during the 12 month study period.

All had histories of previous violence and all but one experienced violence from an early age (H1 and 2). All had had relationship instability (H3) and employment problems (H4). All but one had problems with substance abuse (H5) and all had a major mental illness (H6), the most common being schizophrenia. Although no-one had been formally tested for psychopathy, one person from the original group met criteria for antisocial and borderline personality disorder. All had had developmental trauma, including having been in care from an early age, three had reported having experienced being sexually abused in childhood around the age of nine to ten. All had left school at a mean age of 15.2 years with a mean IQ of 76 (H7, 8 and 9). All were under the Mental Health Act either Section 3 or Section 37/41 with significant family psychiatric histories and medical histories including clozapine induced myocarditis, clozapine induced cardiomyopathy and biventricular failure, neuroleptic malignant syndrome, frontal atrophy, ischemic heart disease, respiratory failure, diabetes and obesity. The mean Brief Psychiatric Rating Scale (BPRS) on admission was 63.

Are we safe?

All staff have completed the Therapeutic Management of Aggression and Violence (TMAV) and/or Personal Safety Training and 100% of staff have completed Security Induction and Security Training. There are an average of 200 patient searches per month, averaging 17 per person and an average of six room searches per month and three random drug tests per patient each month.

There have been no deaths and no escapes. There were seven assaults on staff members over the 12 month time period, (less than one a month) with only one patient-to-patient assault and one absconsion over the same time period, rare events which happen about once a year. There were on average 1.3 episodes of de-escalation per month with an average of one hour spent in de-escalation per month. For the April 2009 to March 2010 period, there was 0.4 episodes of seclusion per month with an average time spent in seclusion of 1.2 hours. No staff took sick leave due to work related violence during the 12 month period.

Unit atmosphere

Michaela has tried to provide high quality involvement in order to deliver a high quality care environment where people are valued as people. Colours and furnishings are carefully chosen to reflect a warmth and to extend a feeling of being cared for, valued and respected. There are house plants, cushions, table cloths and bone china for the visitor and children's lounges. Trying to think about those factors that might be able to be easily quantified, we decided to look at the amount of times the men spent on activities.

'As required' medication was used on 11 occasions in the 12 month period, most often with one man who had a manic relapse.

Leave

Leave status varies as a function of approval from the Ministry of Justice, staff availability to accompany men on escorted leave as well as the person's wellbeing and the lack of incidents for which leave may have been temporarily suspended in order to reassess risk. Each named nurse kindly trawled through the old notes and leave forms for the time period. The data for six patients, (not every named nurse was excited by this request!) revealed an average of 14 escorted and 16 unescorted leaves per month per person. Combined, this means each of the men got out on average every day. The key performance indicators that were developed by the Trust for the commissioners did identify the absolute number of leaves. For eight months of the study period, there were 953 escorted and 1888 unescorted leaves which averages out to 119 and 236 per month respectively. Combined this is 355 leaves per month, or just over ten per day. Interestingly the two approaches at quantifying leave seemed to roughly correspond.

It is difficult at times to provide more leave particularly when two escorts are required for some of the men, at least initially. Staff leave, sickness and training create additional difficulties in staffing.

Clinical outcomes

In addition to the suite of measures we are slowly incorporating on a routine basis, individualised clinical outcomes were instructive. For three of our men the most important outcome was their ability to move on from having become institutionalised. Of the 12 original men, all but one has left. Over a six to 12 month period for the three men for whom the BPRS was relevant, the average of 63 fell to 32.

It has been interesting going through the first 11 men admitted to the unit. The context is important here. I was trained and practised elsewhere and therefore have been less influenced by a UK culture which was risk averse. Looking at the 11 men during the time period April 2009 to March 2010, eight of the men had schizophrenia, two had a personality disorder and one had a bipolar affective disorder. On average the men spent just under one and a half years on Bowman Unit. Interestingly, the majority, eight out of 11 were discharged during this time period. When we look at that group, those who had successfully left had the following features in common; three were on clozapine and four were on depot medication. All had been able to cease or significantly moderate their alcohol and drug intake, had become somewhat involved in activities on the unit, but perhaps more importantly, were discharged to a setting where ongoing support was possible. In particular, three went to our open rehabilitation unit, Fettle House, from which one person has moved on to a supported accommodation house. Three were discharged directly to supported accommodation and three to the community, two of whom had been able to rebuild contact with their family. The other man lived independently but in a series of four units in which a support person visited occasionally and was accessible if further support was required.

With four new admissions, our clinical expectation suggests similar results, albeit with a shorter average length of stay. This will be about six months for three of the men but longer for the person with a solvent induced acquired brain injury and with an inability to recognise the adverse effects of their continued drug and alcohol use leading to protracted hospitalisation.

One man with a 35 year history of institutional care for an intractable personality and one whose psychosis significantly deteriorated were both returned to a medium secure setting. The third man went to Fettle, rehabilitation unit and although remained clinically well from his schizophrenia and free from drugs and alcohol, began to return to his exploitation and intimidation of vulnerable others. Despite a four month trial he had to return to Bowman Unit and individual occupancy accommodation options are being explored.

Psychological understanding of people

As we mentioned above, numbers are important and these numbers are very rough and ready. As such they identify the need to collect this information routinely and systematically as we move to developing a research capability of Bowman under the leadership of Dr Ian Hogbin, our new psychologist. However, there is another way of thinking about outcomes. One of the things which has been important and possible because of the culture Michaela has developed on the unit, is an ability to think about the person. We want to demonstrate this by briefly describing two of our new men, each from two different perspectives. Both are important.

Mikael was referred to us with the possibility of both schizophrenia and an obsessive compulsive disorder. The former was characterised by him receiving persecutory messages through the wall and of hearing birds singing words. He also had an obvious deterioration from his premorbid, university level of functioning. The latter included both aggressive and sexual thoughts which not only frightened and alarmed him, but also the community in which these occurred prior to his hasty admission. The community forensic team had been involved but after a four month admission on a general adult ward, progress had plateaued with an incomplete response to medication and psychological treatments and he was referred to our unit. Initially we too became involved in attempting to delineate whether there were one or two disorders, and to sequentially and methodically treat both separately and then in combination.

He arrived on Bowman from another general adult unit in which it was difficult to respond to incidents in the same way a well staffed low secure unit, orientated specifically around safety, was able to. Within hours of arriving he had upturned the table in the dining room. immediately he was in de-escalation. Rather than accepting this as in response to the psychotic phenomenon he described at the time, he was subsequently able to acknowledge his surprise at how swiftly people moved and in contrast to the unit he had come from and how this made him feel safe. He too had been wondering where the boundaries were.

We then began to notice a pattern; initial progress and then return to 'square one'. It was in reflective practice that Vanessa enabled us to see maybe we too had become paralysed by the risks rather than the realities. The reality of those risks, which included him running into traffic and actually ended up being injured and of his aggressive and sexualised thoughts and actions, which had led to immediate police involvement. If we were too frightened to support him with escorted leave, then we might unwittingly confirm his fears that such thoughts are dangerous. What we as a team had to do was to contain our own anxieties and whilst mindful of risk, neither be paralysed by, or fail to consider, those risks but to support him nevertheless.

We also began to piece together other aspects of his presentation from his life story. His step-brother, with whom he had had a conflictual relationship, was accidentally killed in traffic. We wondered whether at this young age, with the remnants of the magical thinking of childhood, he might have wished his brother was dead. Tragedy struck. What remained seared into his unconscious mind was that thoughts and feelings are dangerous. As he reached adolescence, when aggressive and sexual thoughts emerge, he became too frightened to explore these. Instead he presented to mental health services, initially with non-specific anxiety and depressive symptoms, and then symptoms typical of schizophrenia which gave him an explanation for conflict and distress. The obsessive component was an attempt at controlling these thoughts and feelings. However, while initially medicalised, the lack of a sustained improvement following effective treatments for each disorder, raised the possibility of a negative therapeutic reaction and psychological understanding his presentation. Mikael has now settled, the tension has gone and he has returned home.

The second example we want to write about is Robert who was in his 50s and had schizophrenia. He had come to the attention of the police following numerous and multiple complaints that he was being stalked, and Calor gas was being put into his room and black powder mixed with cocaine in vast quantities into his car. The latter resultied in a serious car accident when he attempted to flee from his persecutors. He eventually accumulated multiple aliases and different dates of birth as he moved around the country for similar reasons. He complained repeatedly, with an unsuccessful hearing at the High Court for inaction on the part of the police. He sought sanctuary in psychiatric unit for a period of two years at which point he believed he would become ordained as a priest and would move to France. Previous attempts at medication had been unsuccessful.

Looking at his story from another perspective, it transpired he was the youngest in a family where his father had been abusive, ('wicked') while his mother was 'good, clean and hard working'. He felt no-one, including the police, had been there to protect him. As an isolated man he eventually met a woman and fell in love with her and from his account, she with him. Three weeks later he saw her in a car with another man and was deeply hurt. He believed she was a 'prostitute' and like the man with her, was 'wicked'. We hypothesised that as the 'good' person, he would not have been able to manage feelings of anger which may have amounted to murderous rage. Nor could he have fallen in love with someone who was 'bad'. We wondered whether he had turned these thoughts around, 'I was never in love with you, it was you who was in love with me' and hence his persistent complaint of stalking. Similarly, 'I couldn't possibly be so angry I would want to kill you, it is you who wish to kill me' and therefore his belief he was being persecuted.

For a long time I wondered about such psychological musings. We have included them not because we believe such psychological understanding might 'cure' in Freud's cathartic sense, rather it enables us to reconnect or remain connected to the person who may also have a psychiatric diagnosis. It is this willingness and openness to consider different aspects of the same person which Michaela has incorporated into the culture of the unit and has continued to develop in Reflective Practice. It is this continued return to each of us as people, of being individuals and of having our own stories that in sense contributes to hopefulness, and to the unit atmosphere. We believe being able to develop a psychological understanding of the person has been one of the most important outcomes for this unit.

What does this cost?

Again it was difficult to know how best to measure this. Dawn, our modern matron, commented 'Bowman Unit's budget was set prior to its opening in January 2008. It was based on providing 12 low secure unit beds at 94% occupancy. Although staffing levels are on the low side compared to other units, the overall cost per bed per day is on the higher side due to our private finance initiative (PFI) contracting arrangements. Comparing costs per low secure unit bed per day 'like for like' feels an impossible task.

In 2009, we increased bed capacity to 14 without any investment into the service and without any detriment to our men. This has made the service more cost-effective and has generated additional income for the Trust by selling the additional beds at the national tariff rate.

For the time period studied, we were on budget, despite a series of discharges occurring and whilst waiting for Ministry of Justice approval for transfers and therefore new admissions.

The other interesting thing about the cost was the

number of additional staff hours used. It averaged out to 1271 hours per month. Quality, at least as expressed in activities, takes money. I am reminded of the Oregon group who suggested there are three aspects to any mental health service: quality, accessibility and cost; choose any two. That is, you can have quality and accessibility but it costs money. The corollary is also important to understand. If you wish to save on costs, than either quality or accessibility suffers.

Captain James Cook and the fight against scurvy

Before finishing this chapter, we wanted to quote from an article entitled 'Disseminating Innovations in Healthcare' published in the Journal of the American Medical Association in 2003 (Vol 289; pages 1969 to 1975).

"As it happens, healthcare is in good company in being slow to use new knowledge. Diffusion of innovation is, after all, a challenge in many human enterprises. The history of the treatment of scurvy shows how variable diffusion can be.

For many centuries, scurvy was the main threat to the health of naval crews. When Vasco de Gama sailed around the Cape of Good Hope for the first time in 1497, 100 of his crew of 160 men died of scurvy. Nobody knew about vitamin C at that time, but some dietary factor was suspected. Captain James Lancaster proved it in 1601, when commanding a fleet of four ships on a voyage from England to India. On that voyage, the crew on one ship were given three teaspoons of lemon juice every day. At the half-way point on the trip, 110 (40%) of 278 sailors on the other three ships had died of scurvy, but none died on the ship with the lemon juice rations.

However, no-one seemed to notice; despite Lancaster's evidence, practices in the British Navy did not change. The study was repeated 146 years later in 1747 by a British Navy Physician named James Lind. In a random trial of six treatments for scorbutic sailors on HMS Salisbury, citrus again proved effective against scurvy. It still took the British Navy 48 more years to react by ordering that citrus fruit became part of the diet on all navy ships. Scurvy in the British Navy disappeared altogether almost overnight. The British Board of Trade took 70 more years to adopt the innovation, ordering a proper diet on merchant marine vessels in 1865. The total time elapsed from Lancaster's definitive study to universal British preventive policy on scurvy was 264 years".

Wow! We have been heartened by this story for the following reasons. It took 264 years to successfully prevent and treat a disease with a 40% mortality rate. Whenever we try and introduce change, we are reassured if we are able to do so in a time frame of less than 264 years, then we are doing okay. It kind of takes the pressure off!

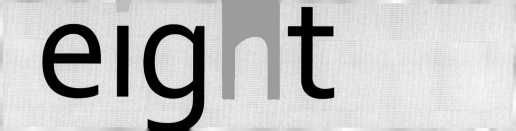

A cartoon from Mr A

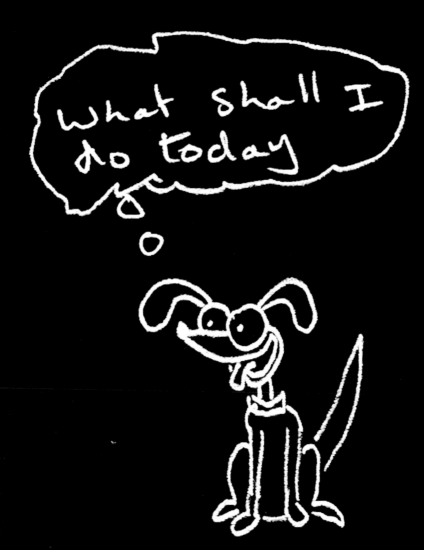

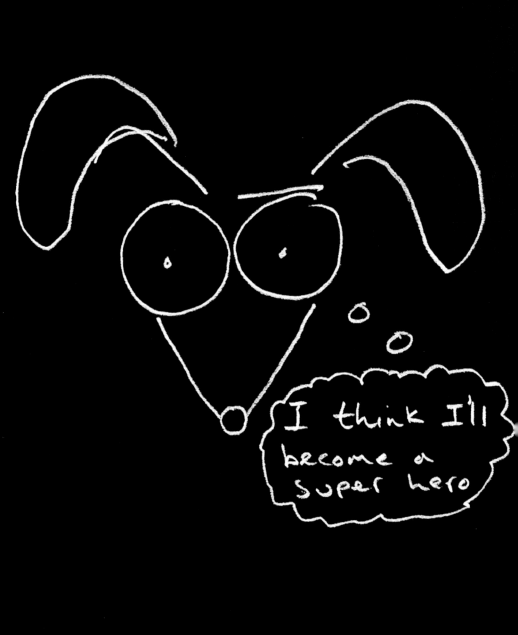

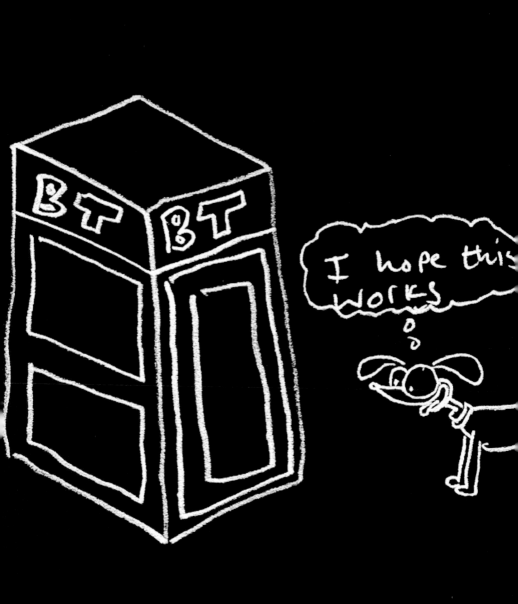

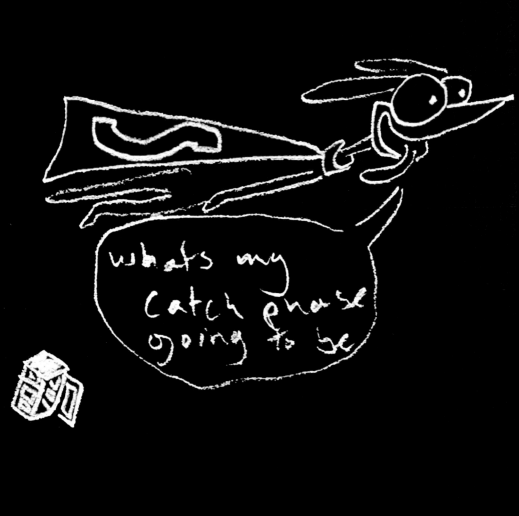

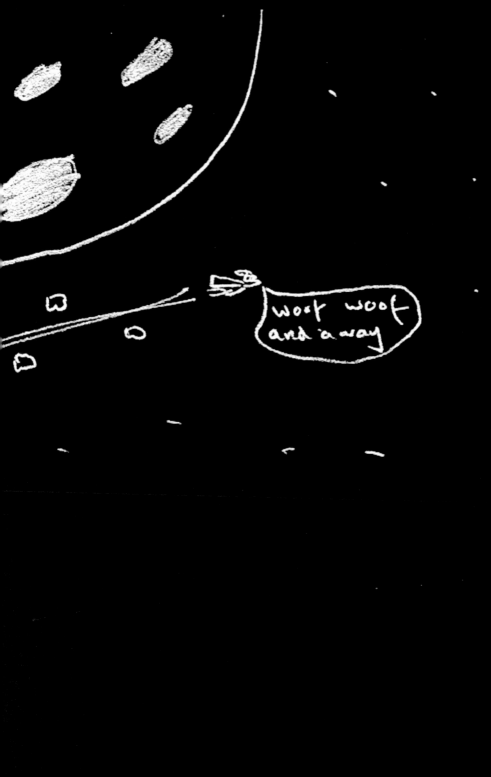

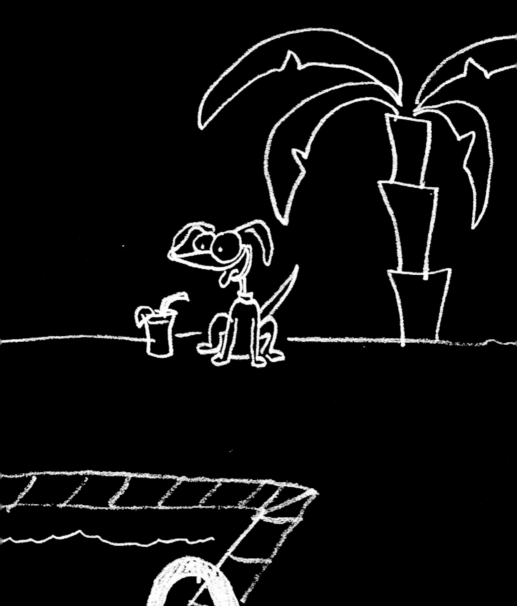
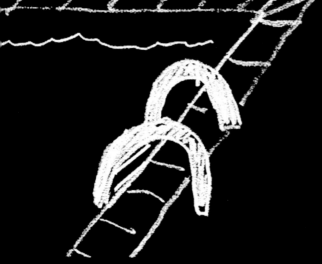

24 The people who make it possible

Here's the Team

Gary Andrews

Elizabeth Baxter

Michaela Burt

Catriona Canning

Vicky Coles

Lynn Corps

Godwim Datip

Chris Dawe

Pete Donegan

William Fearnley

Becky Fox

Brian Hellings

Lee Herman

Ian Hogbin

Christine Jardine

Iain Knox

Wendy Lawry

John Little

Siva Appan

Blix

Raymond Buscombe

Ian Carr

Jackie Conium

Annette Crawford

Luke Davis

Joyce Done

Ian Edgerton

Mark Featherston

Lisa Francey

Rebecca Hepples

Karen Higgins

Gerry Jackson

Jeanette Jenkins

Hannah Lapham

Becky Lewis

Peter Long

Russell Lutchman	Sarah Mably
Birgit Maher	Karen Masters
Phil McNamara	Siobhan Monaghan
Rosina Moore	Dave Pearce
Tim Moore	Sarah Prout
Perry Savage	Gill Searle
Marianne Seebold	Matthew Sharpe
Carol Steward	Gary Swann
Mandy Taylor	Adrian Towler
Pearl Vigus	Annabel Walmsley
Jess Watkins	Tony Whelan
Ian Wotherspoon	Glynn Williams

Thanks!

References

We didn't want to include a series of references for this book, there being excellent text books available which do this task better than we might. However we thought it might be useful to bring to the attention of the interested reader some of those books and articles we found particularly helpful as we went along. As we listed them, we also became aware they too told a story.

Articles:

'The Corruption of Care' The Ely Hospital Enquiry 1969, In: Scandal, social policy and social welfare, Butler and Drakeford, Chapter 3 by J Wardhaugh and P Wilding: Critical Social Policy, 1993, 13: 4-31: Towards an explanation of the corruption of care

Alongside the Ely Inquiry report, this was interesting reading. It gave me a sense of why there needs to be regular reviews, audits and changes that at times seem additional, obvious and unnecessary intrusions into clinical practice.

Counter transference Hate in the Treatment of Suicidal Patients by John Maltsberger and D Buie: Archives of General Psychiatry, 1974; 30: 625-633

Difficult to read and I am still not sure that I necessarily understand all parts of it.

However, I have found it useful to re-read on a number of occasions noting in particular the latter part of the article which describes the various defensive positions we take up. The ability to be able to become aware of those for ourselves and to talk about them is important in our work.

The Treatment of Antisocial Syndromes: The Therapist's Feelings by Larry Strasberger: In: Unmasking the Psychopath, W H Reid (ed), W W Norton & Co, pp 191-207, 1986

This article, which we mentioned in the chapters above, explores specific issues that may arise when working with someone who meets criteria for Antisocial Personality Disorder.

Assessing and Managing the Risks of Violence Towards Others, Paul Mullen and James Ogloff In: Oxford Textbook of Psychiatry (2nd Edition) M Gelder (Ed)

Paul Mullen always writes in a thoughtful and scholarly fashion, this piece is no exception. As I used to say to

Registrars, "It doesn't matter what he's talking about, just go!"

"Simply to be let in": Inclusion as a basis of recovery, Psychiatric Rehabilitation Journal, 2001; 24: 375-388

I liked this article and although a bit repetitive, it did serve to remind me that in order to manage my own anxiety, I have at times felt I needed to get the person completely well before contemplating leave or inclusion in activities on the unit and in the community. As the article points out, this is unreasonable as it is for others who may not recover including the blind, the hard of hearing and amputees. As a society, we have adapted the environment that enables people to be included.

The Myth of The Hero Innovator and Alternative Strategies for Organisational Change by Nicholas Georgiades, Lyndon Phillimore In: Behaviour Modification with the Severely Retarded Kiernan, Woodford (ed), 1975

I think their quote says it quite nicely, namely "The future of the matter is that organisations such as schools and hospitals will, like dragons, eat hero innovators for breakfast." The article then goes on to describes ways in which the job may be shared while acknowledging the difficulties that are inevitably attached.

Disseminating Innovations in Health Care by Donald Berwick, Journal of the American Medical Association, 2010; 289: 1969-1975

This follows on from the Hero Innovator and it looks at and describes those in the organisation who embrace new ideas early on, those who like to wait and see and those who find it difficult to adopt change, recognising this as being part of human nature. Quite useful.

Biology is important:

The Prefrontal Cortex: a target for antipsychotic drugs by F Artigas: Acute Psychiatrist Scandinavia, 2010; 121: 11-21

I came across this article recently and whilst I don't begin to understand the biological technicalities, it is part of the emerging literature that has sought to link biological underpinnings to psychosocial circumstances, behaviour and pharmacological intervention. It will be interesting to see how this develops over time and again is as much about keeping the hope alive as it is about hard and fast facts.

Medication Treatment of Different Types of Alcoholism by B A Johnson, American journal of Psychiatry, 2010; 167, 630-670

As with the above, this was another interesting read and

with developments and an approach that encourages a sure footing and restores hope.

Pharmacotherapy for Borderline Personality Disorder: Cochrane systematic review of randomised trials by Lieb et al: British Journal of Psychiatry, 2010; 196, 4-12

Similar and interesting that psychopharmacology is becoming interested in a disorder where people really do struggle.

Acute Antipsychotic Induced Akathisia Revisited by M Poyurovsky: British Journal of Psychiatry 2010; 196: 89-91

Interesting again how old problems when re-visited may suggest previously unthought of options.

We would be interested if you had other books or references you have found particularly useful in order that we may share amongst the field.

Books:

Enabling Recovery: The principles and practice of rehabilitation psychiatry, edited by Glen Roberts, Sarah Davenport, Frank Holloway, Theresa Tattan: Gaskell, The Royal College of Psychiatrists, London, 2006

Not surprisingly, this was a highly recommended text by the Royal College of Psychiatrists. It is a very readable up-to-date and very much a positive and recovery focused text book on rehabilitation and psychiatry.

It's got lots of sections you can easily dip into and we found it a very useful foundation text for our unit.

Psychiatric Intensive Care edited by Dominic Beer, Stephen Percira and Carol Paton: Greenwich Medical Media, London, 2010

This text was written largely with the Psychiatric Intensive Care Unit in mind, although the chapters on Seclusion, Restraint and Psychological Approaches to Long-Term Patients were helpful and thoughtful.

An Integrated Approach to Family Work for Psychosis by Gina Smith, Karl Gregory and Annie Higgs: Jessica Kingsley Publishers, London, 2007

As to family work, I wasn't quite sure what to do other than just jumping in and having a bit of a go and seeing what happened.

I found this manual for family work very readable. It is down to earth and useful as background information for what is quite a specialised area. We are certainly grateful for the recent involvement of our family intervention service.

The Psychopathic Mind: Ongoing, dynamic treatment by J Reid Meloy, 1988

I have referred to this in one of the chapters, and along with one of the articles that I mention below, found it thoughtful and useful in coming to terms with the strong reactions that arise when working with people with antisocial personality disorder.

A Practical Guide to Forensic Psychotherapy edited by Estelle V Welldon and Cleo Van Velsen: Jessica Kingsley publishers, London, 1997

Again I found this useful in continuing to find ways of bringing a psychologically orientated approach to a chronic unit where progress may be slow or risks may be personal and the possibility of untoward reactions spilling out in unhelpful ways

The Relationship Management of the Borderline Patient by David Dawson and Harriet Macmillan: Rutledge, Taylor and Francis Group, New York, 1993

Without doubt this remains the most useful orientation towards working with people with borderline personality disorder I have found.

It adopts quite a different approach from the traditional. However being able to change tack and to work alongside the person, each trying to do their bit as responsible and competent adults, makes a difference.

Manic Depressive Illness: Bipolar disorders and recurrent depression (2nd Edition) by Fred Goodwin and Kay Wilhelm: Oxford University Press, New York, 2007

While the majority of our clinical population had chronic schizophrenia, there have been on occasion those individuals who have been hospitalised for seemingly intractable, rapid cycling bipolar affective disorder.

Fred Goodwin's text is encyclopaedic in its breadth and depth. I found it particularly useful in being able to read about aspects of care and the detail of the text which afforded clinical and therapeutic opportunities and therefore hope.

Stahl's Essential Psychopharmacology: Neuroscientific basis and practical application (3rd Edition) by Steven Stahl: Cambridge University Press, New York, 2008

Although this is an American text with an unashamed polypharmacy approach to the major mental illnesses, it did provide at least a theoretic rationale for trialling new agents and/or combinations of agents. Where these pan-out in reality is perhaps less important than retaining focus and hope for people.

The Importance of Disappointment by I Craib: Routlege, 1994

An interesting little book that I found in my predecessor's library. It was quite useful as it reminded me of the reality of what we are doing captured perhaps in the comment "Life is not like this all of the time, but it is like this some of the time."

Schizophrenia is a Human Process by Harry Stack Sullivan: W W Norton & Co, New York, 1962

I'm a bit nervous about including this title for as I went to search for it, I noticed its reference to psychoanalysis and schizophrenia. The name Harry Stack Sullivan had always intrigued me and I remembered it from my psychology days where psychoanalysis was heavily criticised. I decided to include it although I can't say I understood all of it. What impressed me though was Sullivan's ability to sit with people who remained floridly psychotic as he attempted to understand what they might be trying to say amidst their abnormal beliefs and thought disorder. Remarkable and important particularly as many of our men have not responded to multiple medications.

It is funny that when particular pieces come along we are not always in a place to appreciate them. Others acquire new meaning when read again. We hope these help and if you come across other little gems, you pass them on.

nine

Appendices

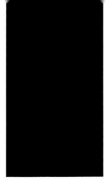

Appendix 1

Minutes of Community Meeting
Thursday 30 April 2009 at 09:30

Issues:

1. Cigarette lighters

    Discussion: Further to our earlier community meeting where this matter had been addressed, there have been a small number of individuals who forget or fall asleep or for other reasons haven't handed in their cigarette lighters prior to going to bed. This leaves the staff in the unpleasant situation of having to wake and remind those persons.

    The discussion also included the notion that those individuals who did remember may be unfairly penalised if all lighters were removed.

    Consensus: What was generally agreed was three non-consecutive strikes for a given individual would result in their cigarette lighter being returned to the staff for an as yet undefined period of time, at which point a further opportunity in testing responsibility could be offered.

2. Violent and Pornographic Material on the Unit

    Discussion: Interestingly, importantly and thankfully there was no person who was suggesting that violent and/or explicit pornographic material should be available on the unit at any time.

    Difficulties were expressed in terms of what might be regarded as 'too violent', the difficulty in distinguishing between old war films and horror movies; magazines such as 'FHM, Zoo' and 'lingerie models' were ok.

    Individual differences, and again, trust and responsibility by each of those individuals was raised. This arose in the context of potential internet access, individual televisions in each person's bedroom should this occur in the future.

    A view was expressed that no violent or sexually explicit material should be available at any time.

    Consensus: Interestingly there appeared to be a similar theme developing, namely related to the notion of trust and personal responsibilities, each individual being 'grown up' about it. Again this could be monitored and if there were untoward events arising out of any of the above, the matter could be reconsidered with that particular individual.

3. The suggestion of having one of the rooms on the unit converted to a sensory room

    Discussion: The matter was raised and thought to be a good idea.

4. Thanks were expressed to those who assisted in the relocation of the garden shed and the compost, including those who just wanted to come out and have a look at what was going on!

5. Where we as a community felt on the 'too soft through to too hard' spectrum. Particularly as new people are likely to be arriving on the unit, the theme noted above was again evident. Namely that we begin to trust and become responsible for our actions, we know what is unacceptable, that it is important to be sensitive to others who may have different views and that again we are 'grown up about it'.

    If things work 'ok' then we continue this as a guiding principal to our community. If it doesn't work out for whatever reason, then this leads to exploration, understanding and revision of those decisions. The opinion again appeared to emerge of regarding people as 'responsible and competent' and use that as a starting framework.

6. Hygiene and Cleanliness

    Discussion: The observation that the courtyard was sometimes left littered; jobs on the rota were not being done; coffee cups were often not available or dirty. Further, that some people do what is required but others are not doing this.

    There was a general agreement that 'it had gone slack again' and that this was an ongoing issue that needed to be managed.

    Various suggestions were made including an offer of all to develop a new rota. However to have this role designated to a specific individual may leave them the target of unfair criticism.

    A suggestion was made that each person has their own named cup with a further suggestion of plastic or wooden spoons for stirring.

    The issue extended to the availability of milk and the observation that residents have at times taken other people's milk and food. For people who have no more leave this is difficult. It was also noted that it can be difficult to challenge someone or to say 'no' when asked whether or not they can use another person's foodstuff as it can be to approach staff.

Consensus: It was decided that this topic should be discussed in the next community meeting.

That again it was another example around individuals taking responsibility.

It was difficult to know quite how to monitor and manage jointly agreed sanctions unless this was done on an individual basis.

Minutes of Community Meeting
Thursday 10 September 2009

Issues:

1. Activities for the Day

   Dr Little had no idea about this. Left it until then end of the meeting, couldn't find the paperwork and when he did it was from yesterday. Still, it was a sunny day!

2. Hourly Checks

   Discussion: Hourly observations are required as part of providing a safe and secure unit. However the staff have also become aware that this can be troublesome, particularly at night.

   Some discussion was had regarding this with suggestions that staff could knock, call the person's name and wait for a reply. Suggestion was made for a smaller torch or one of those blue LED torches in order to avoid shining a full beam into a person's face. Others preferred that the shutters were opened and that the staff member could look in rather than knock and that this in particular should occur after 22:00.

Privacy arose in relation to this with one person in particular acknowledging that he is not going to be undressed in the area through which the staff can look through the shutters and made the additional useful comment that, as with other parts of our unit philosophy, monitoring is individualised.

Consensus: After 22:00 people would prefer a visual check rather than a knock on the door, that a smaller torch be used and that named nurses discuss with their individual patient what they would prefer and that this is placed on the door for other staff to adhere to.

3. Alcohol

    Discussion: Men were invited to contribute to Bowman developing an approach towards alcohol and that there was going to be a meeting planned for Thursday 8th October at 09:30 with comments and contributions being welcomed.

    The issue was around whether to provide

opportunities to test alcohol use whilst attached to the unit and how that might occur. The matter has arisen recently given the revocation of leave for two of the men who recently drank whilst on unescorted leave.

Experiences from other units were noted including a pub group on the afternoon, that Fettle House allows something like two cans of beer on the unit one night a week in a social setting and wondered whether or not that could be introduced on to Bowman, and that other units have allowed a shandy or a pint out at the pub.

Dr Little expressed his reservations about having alcohol on the unit given that we are a low secure setting. Maintaining this approach, the possibility of freer access on Fettle provides an incentive to become part of the Bowman programme in order that progress to Fettle may be made.

Again the notion of individually assessing and managing risk was raised with some individuals for whom alcohol is a significant problem and who may require life long abstention, whereas others might be able to have 'a controlled drinking programme' whereby there is an experience of going to and enjoying a pub without alcohol, with a shandy or with a maximum of one pint; and of those being with a meal. Similarly, supervision should be tailored to the individual rather than a blanket institutionalised rule.

When it came to the consequences for breaches of leave opportunities, 7 days loss of all leave for the first occasion, 1 month for the second and 3 to 6 months for the third occasion seemed to be reasonably balance consequences from becoming overly restrictive or punitive. This acknowledges that if this is an identified area of difficulty for a person, then it is an area that requires work on how to help that person manage an identified problem that limits their ability to move forward.

4. Volunteers

Discussion: On Tuesday 15th September at 09:30, Terry from Truro and his Bodmin equivalent, Christine, are coming to the unit meeting at the above time and will hopefully attended by Sarah our Social Inclusion Worker.

Terry runs Volunteer Cornwall and was first approached with the possibility of providing volunteers that would enable greater escorted leave, particularly when staff numbers are low. However Terry also has a number of other services available, including the possibility of us volunteering and helping others. It is a funny thing but when we give, we get.

5. Violent Videos

    Discussion: As with items 2 and 3, this also engendered considerable discussion.

    In particular, the distinction between action movies such as 'Judgement Day' and 'Terminator' were seen as distinctly different from horror and violence as evidenced in videos such as 'Friday 13th', some of the new video games with blood being splattered were all seen as 'a bit much'. The observation was made that the Hungerford massacre was spurred on by the person having seen the 'Rambo' movies a hundred times.

    The observation was also made that the pendulum shouldn't swing the other way, namely with only access to cartoons whereby people are inadvertently made to feel like children.

    The suggestion was made about none of the above movies being suitable for the communal area and the question arising as to whether we as a unit should restrict certain movies. Again the replies were both interesting and important. In particular decisions should be individualised and if there are specific people with specific problems, then this needs to be thought about and managed appropriately. The second interesting comment, from Jonathan I think, that staff have a strong responsibility to make clear about what is right and what is wrong.

6. Barbecue on Sunday

   Discussion: Hopefully the weather will hold and we will be able to have a barbecue to farewell Paul who has been offered and accepted a place at Parcside, signing his tenancy agreement this week. Congratulations to Paul and we genuinely hope that he will keep in contact with us.

7. Cigarettes and Lighters

   Discussion: Don't! In particular, don't walk up the corridors with a lit cigarette and return lighters before going to bed. The staff don't like having to wake people up and intrude. Equally, I was aware when I was on call the other week that I was asked to see and assess a lady who had dropped a cigarette and set her house on fire. She was admitted to hospital.

Minutes of Community Meeting
Thursday 6th May 2010

Issues:

1. Cornwall's Got Talent

   Thanks for the comments and ideas in preparation for our Away Day later this month where we hope to continue to refine and hopefully improve upon what we do on Bowman.

You men felt that what we did well included being supportive, interacting with patients and feeding you, although not always as much as you would like!

Some of you have been frightened by other men on the unit and some of you don't feel as well as you would like to, finding it difficult to 'get a grip on your lives'.

Go-karting came up as an interest as did the Adrenaline Quay near Liskeard and surfing. This is something that we are aware of when trying to identify activities that are going to be of interest to men. These are often outdoor and adventure activities that are sometimes hard to staff and resource but we take your suggestions on board and thank you for them.

Again from memory from last year, the general feeling was that you felt we had the balance about right with regard to risk taking, neither being too strict or too lax. This is important.

In terms of changes you would like to make on Bowman, there was quite a bit of support for having the garden door open all day in order that you might get up in the morning and just go outside irrespective of the weather. Your feeling was that it was a secure area and with CCTV coverage. We will take this back to our security group.

The only other suggestions you made were in relation to asking people to put cigarettes in the bin provided, rather than flicking them on the ground.

Once again thanks and if you've got any other ideas, please let us know.

Minutes of Community Meeting
Thursday 29th July 2010

Issues:

1. A chaotic feel to the unit

    Just sitting in this morning's meeting I was aware of how people were angry, leaving the meeting and resenting being here.

    Considerable discussion followed with a number of men commenting in particular about Will teasing others, following others, having a go at others, blowing kisses or putting his hands down his pants and overstepping the mark in an attempt to get a reaction. If he is told he won't stop and 'somebody is going to deck him'.

    There was an acknowledgement that it is not always easy living on the unit but we all have to get on together. Various suggestions were made including telling staff, but together the Community Meeting decided that what would be most helpful is for Will to hear this from his peers. Accordingly we thought patients and staff together would sit and talk to Will this afternoon; saying that whilst he is likeable, his present behaviour is causing problems for others.

The other person was distressed at being locked up for no reason was Michael. He reported that he should just be locked up in a room and left with cigarettes or just be let out. He didn't feel that he would change whether he stayed here for one month or six months given the previous experiences that he has had. He added that he had no idea why he was here and when asked was able to comment that he had been 'antisocial' although apart from taking drugs was unclear what he might have been doing that has led to a renewal of his section.

Again men were helpful and genuinely tried to explore suggestions and offer advice including accepting that he is here and try to do what is required, keeping your head down and getting involved, of organising your day, talk to staff, don't stay in bed, keep your room tidy, stay out of trouble. Men also asked whether or not there was anything that Michael himself might like doing, but he was unclear.

Michael continued saying that it was unfair that people make decisions for him and that this drives him to suicide. Again the men were helpful and not alarmed and said that people including his family wouldn't want that to happen and wouldn't let it happen. Again suggestions were made in terms of accepting and getting involved.

2. Camping

   After the recent football match where a London based LSU came down and camped overnight, David made the suggestion for the men doing this locally, including cooking sausages in the outdoors.

   Dr Little thought this would be 'a nightmare' but David persisted and encouraged the staff to think about this as a possibility given that the London LSU was able to do this.

3. Crockery

   We forgot to discuss this, but wonder how people felt about crockery instead of plastic mugs?

   I will try to remember for the next community meeting.

Minutes of Community Meeting
Thursday 12th November 2009

Issues:

1. Welcome to Tom and Daniel

    Dr Little extended a welcome to Tom and Daniel having been away on the previous week when they had arrived.

2. Mark returned to Langdon Hospital

    Sadly Mark became poorly over the last few days. Fortunately Mark recognised this himself and the need for him to return to Langdon Hospital. We look forward to catching up with him there and welcoming him back when he settles and returns to Cornwall which we hope will be in the not too distant future.

3. Thanks extended to Paul G

    Paul was available for the presentation by a psychologist who has applied for the psychologist's job. The team are most grateful for Paul's contribution and thoughtful questioning of the candidate in a respectful and appropriate manner.

    Thanks were also extended to the other men that were asked but were unavailable for various reasons but did consider the request.

4. Reminder of times

Men were reminded that in order to manage the many and varied requests, that requests for money occur at two times during the day at 10:00 and 14:00 and that requests to visit the shop are at 10:00 and 16:00.

5. London meeting

Dr Little reported that last week he attended a two day conference on schizophrenia. As before he wanted to try and communicate information obtained from various conferences.

Whilst a lot of the material was quite detailed and complicated, the bits that I was able to understand included the idea that schizophrenia is an illness that although not necessarily obvious from birth, many people showed difficulties early on. These included being born early, difficulties around birth, being slow to talk and walk as well as having family difficulties, being exposed to drugs, particularly marijuana at an early age and other stressors. The presence of early symptoms that were suggestive but perhaps overlooked that subsequently progressed into a clear picture of schizophrenia in adolescence or in the early twenties was also talked about. Accordingly, schizophrenia has been conceptualised as a 'neurodevelopmental disorder'.

The other thinking around schizophrenia is that

somehow various parts of the brain had not developed normally. There are changes to the surface of the brain and deep within the brain. Particularly around adolescence when various fibres within the brain being pruned, this process is exaggerated and perhaps more haphazard leading to a 'disconnectivity'. That is, through no fault of the person, the wiring of various parts of the brain has been affected. This has a number of potential clinical implications including affecting a person's ability to remember and their ability to judge things correctly or accurately. People with schizophrenia tend to be forgetful, jump to conclusions and have a certain impulsivity with a difficulty in pausing, reflecting and learning from previous mistakes. Marijuana, alcohol and other drugs specifically made this worse.

Unfortunately little of the conference was devoted to treatment. It was interesting to see the research that is combining both biological and environmental or psychosocial treatments. I was quite excited by the possibility of understanding a biological basis to the psychosocial work that Michaela Burt in particular has led and inspired, specifically physical activity in no matter what form to improve motor skills, social activity in whatever form to promote social inclusion and specific projects around thinking skills that we hope to introduce as a refined treatment package that would enable progress through Bowman.

Hopefully we will be able to develop some of these ideas during the next few months and I hope to keep in contact with some of the speakers for this purpose.

Minutes of Community Meeting
Thursday 18th June 2009

Will, Iain and myself attended a conference in London entitled 'Security Issues in Forensic Settings' instead of attending the Community Meeting.

Feedback:

As usual, I wanted to be able to report back to you things that we found to be helpful.

Ministry of Justice:

It was interesting to hear from the Head of the Mental Health Unit giving her perspective of the Ministry of Justice, the audience making a number of complaints the response they had or had not received. Penny was clear that the Case Managers with whom we interact are not clinically trained and are civil servants. She further highlighted the key role that she thought the Ministry of Justice plays, namely to take an impartial view where the most important focus was on safety for the community. In particular she highlighted how effective she thought the Ministry of Justice had been and that this was important ministerally. Additional speakers described the likely development of a Victim's Commissioner with an emphasis much more on the impact on victims and according the safety of the community.

What was clear was that the Ministry of Justice is likely to continue a very cautious and conservative approach towards escorted and unescorted leaves for the foreseeable future.

Low Secure Units

Although the conference was predominantly around forensic hospitals such as Broadmoor and medium secure units, it was useful to see that Bowman as a Low Secure Unit was attending to the same principles related to security of the larger facilities. In particular it would seem that the balance between the physical environment with non-accessible windows and perimeter fence for example, the various procedures that we have in terms of random searches, drug and alcohol screening, monitoring and documenting carefully escorted and unescorted leaves and getting to know individual patients and the relationships that are formed both between patients and staff are all essential parts of providing a secure unit. To this end, we have recently started a reflective group on the unit for the staff to become mindful of subtleties in relationships that might affect our ability to care and provide treatment and accordingly every three weeks, we would ask you as a community to provide us with this time. I will come to the meeting on the next morning that his occurs which should be Monday 13th July at 10:00. I would be grateful for your support in protecting this time for the staff.

Creative Tension

One of the main themes that emerged through the conference was trying to find a balance between being too strict on the one hand and too lacsidasical on the other. Peter, security advisor at HMP Whitemoor was clear that care and clinical work was completely irrelevant and the prime concern should be one of security. Unfortunately he was involved in a shooting of a colleague as an armed group entered the prison and enabled the escape, albeit temporary, of six IRA members. However, the clinical members of the audience were interested in being able to create an environment which enabled people to make use of the work available and to have an opportunity to progress with positive risk taking and graded but cautious progress. It was Bill Abbott, one of the other speakers formally from the Department of Health, who raised the notion of the creative tension that occurs between these two differing positions and that it was each unit's ability to find the balance between security and care. I couldn't help but feel that at Bowman we had a reasonable balance of security and rehabilitative care.

Clever Technology

I'm not particularly technologically competent or interested in becoming so, but did listen to a talk on various emerging technologies to monitor people in the community including Femto Cell Cellular Networks, voice analysis for stress detection, intelligent image processing, biometrics, face recognition and electronic tagging. I have no idea what most of these mean, but can see how they might begin to become part of at least forensic prison practice, if not clinical practice. I'd be interested in your views on being electronically tagged as part of unescorted leave provisions.

Cornwall's Got Talent

Hi Men

To get the most out of our 'Away Day', can you think about, fill out and send this to my secretary Karen in the internal post, but do not put your name on it and Karen will not recognise your handwriting.

We'll collate the replies, including any other matters that you want to raise and discuss on the day.

1.   What do we do well?
2.   What patient groups benefit most from the skills we have?
3.   What are we 'not so good at'?
4.   Have you been frightened at work? How could this be managed differently?
5.   Have you felt frustrated at work? How could this be managed differently?
6.   What interests you? By this we mean what would you like to learn more about when you are working on Bowman?
7.   What gives you job satisfaction on Bowman?
8.   Risk taking – any thoughts?
9.   What changes would you like to make on Bowman?
10. I can't think of a tenth question, can you? (and answer one too!)

We really appreciate your thoughts on this. Bowman is important and we have an opportunity to develop a model in LSU patient care.